Urinary Tract Infection and Nephropathy - Insights into Potential Relationship

Edited by Ran Pang

Published in London, United Kingdom

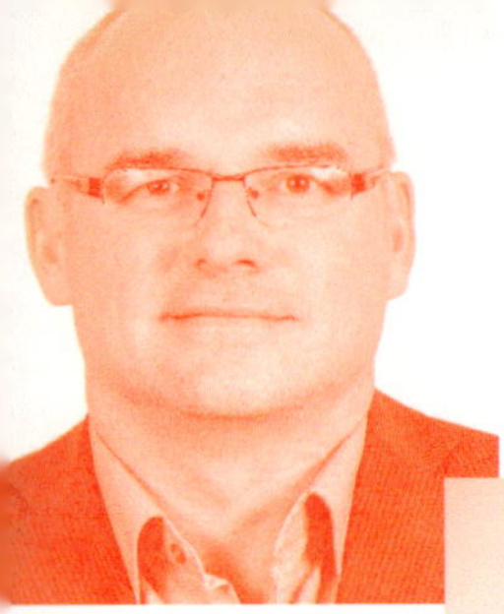
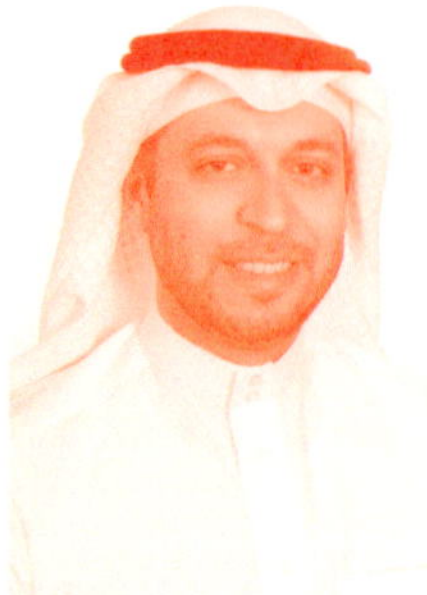
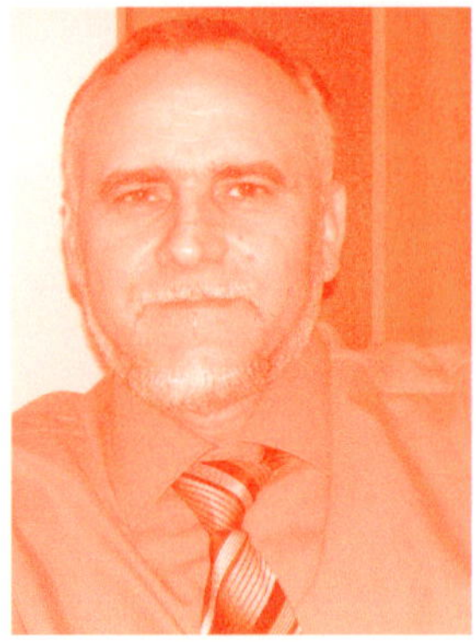
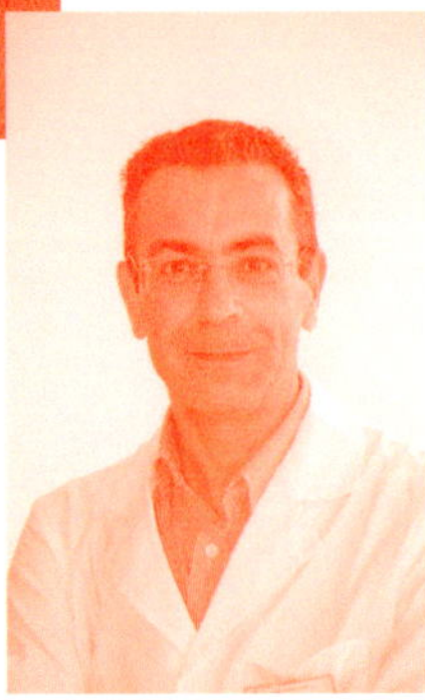
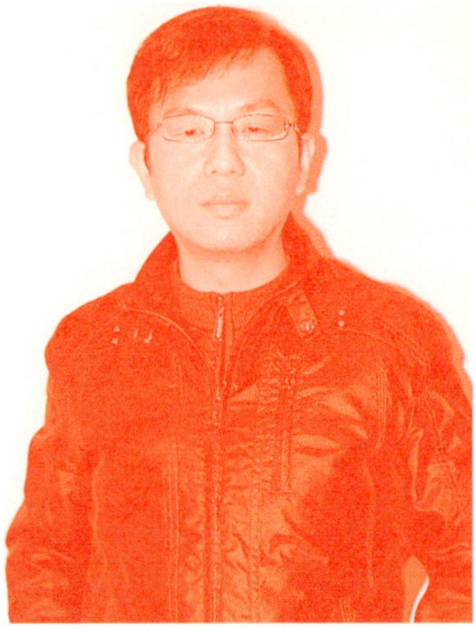
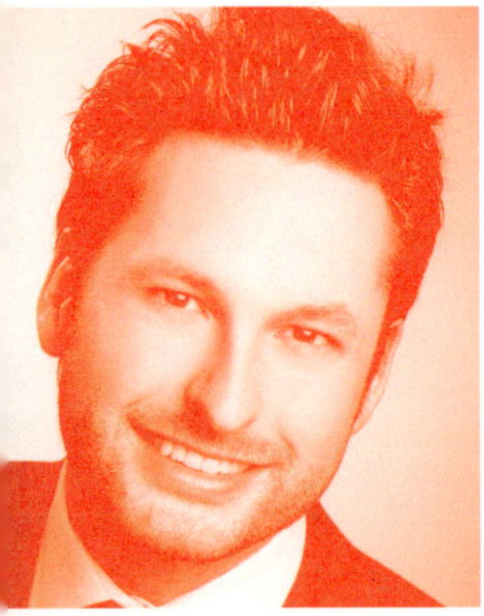
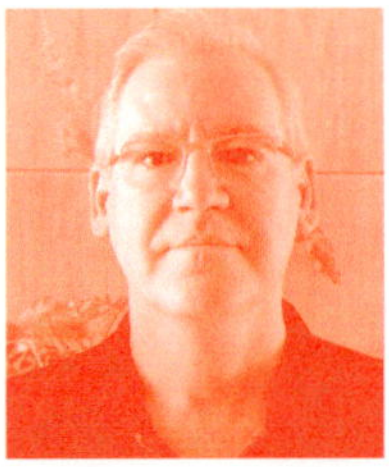

IntechOpen

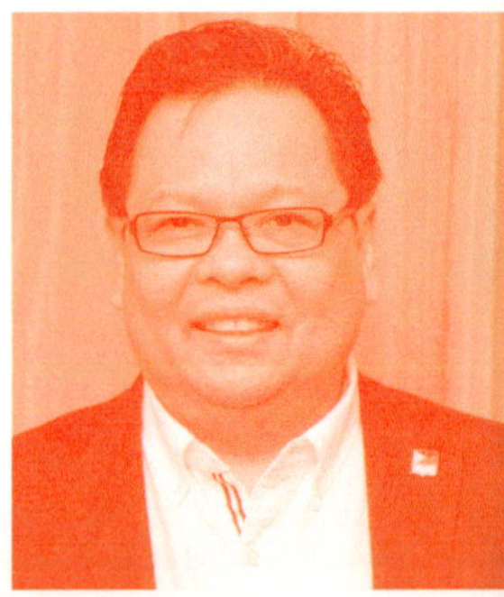
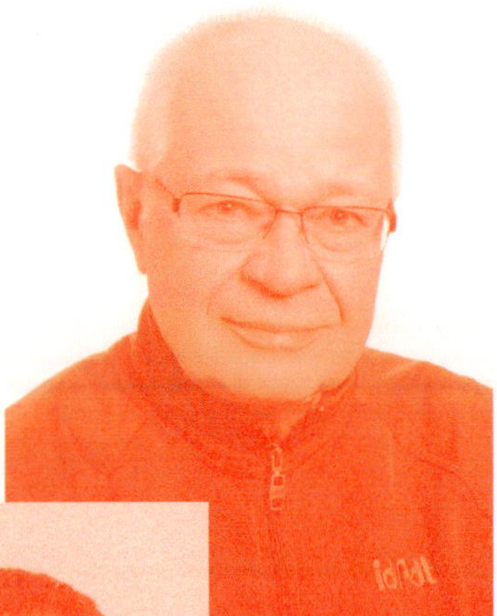
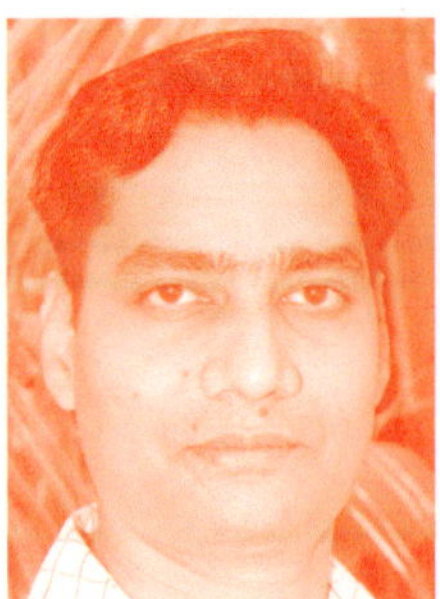
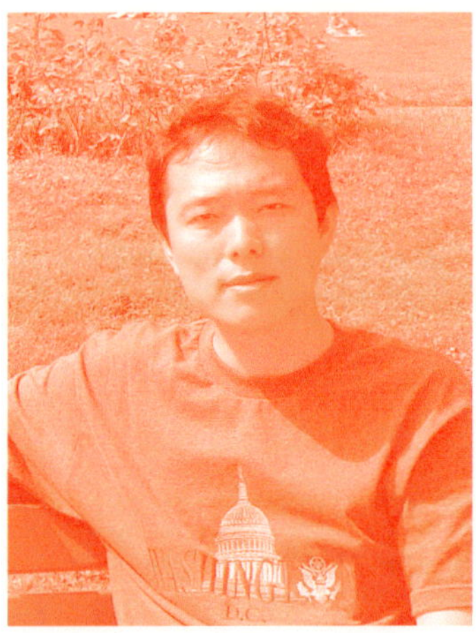
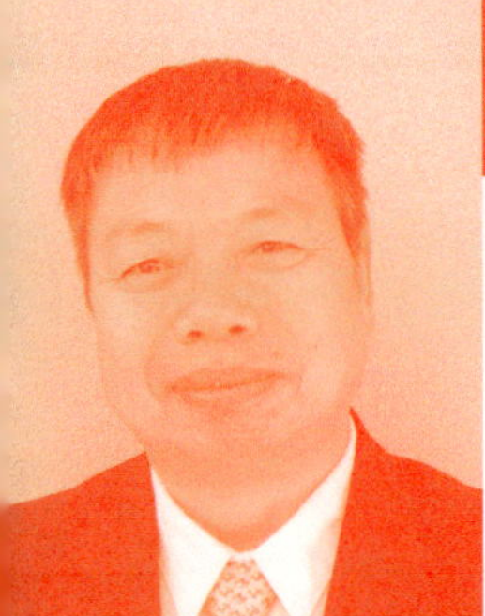
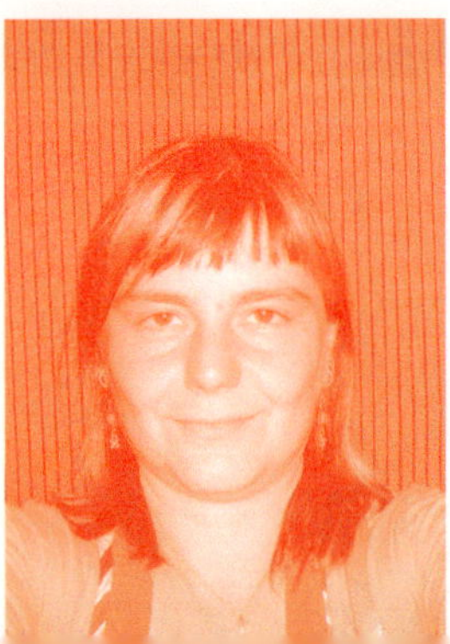

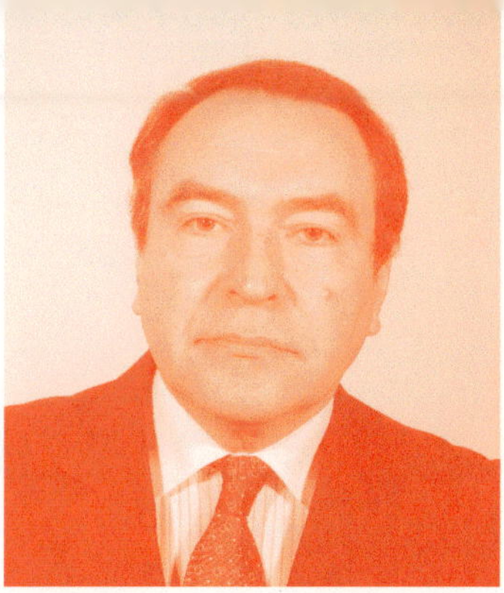
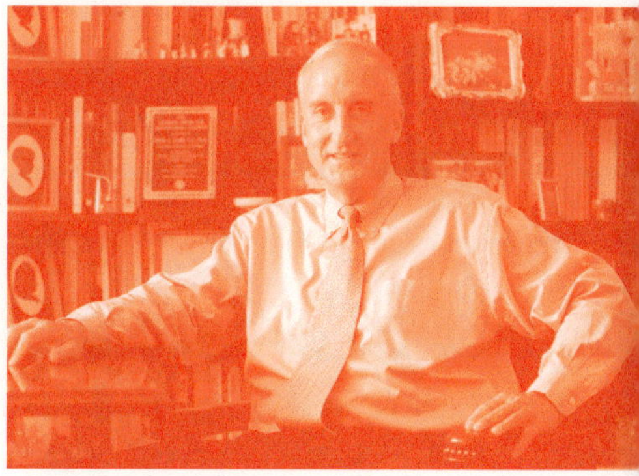
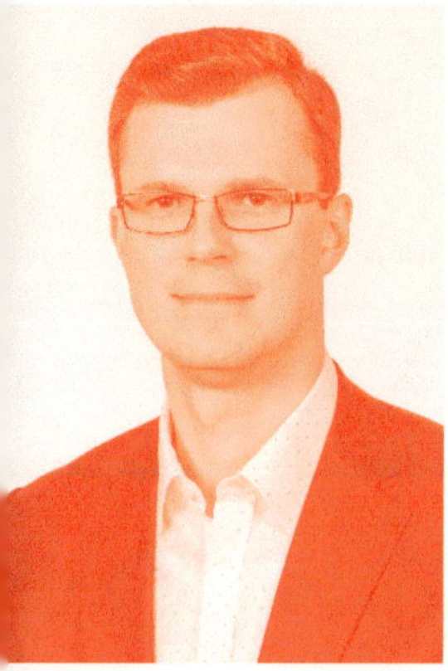
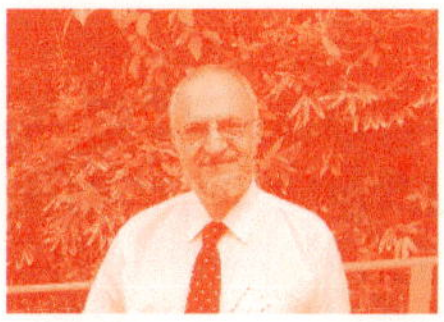
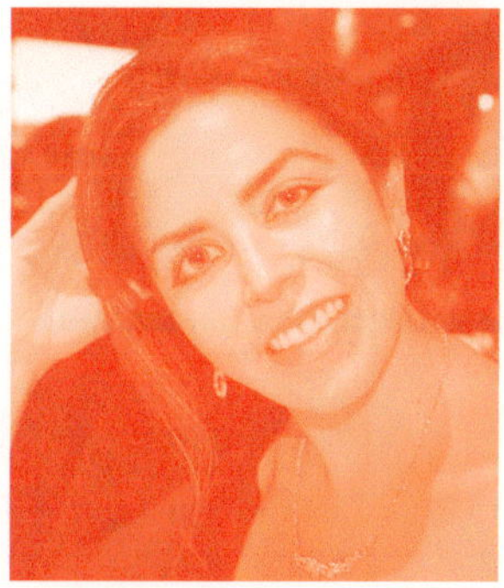

Supporting open minds since 2005

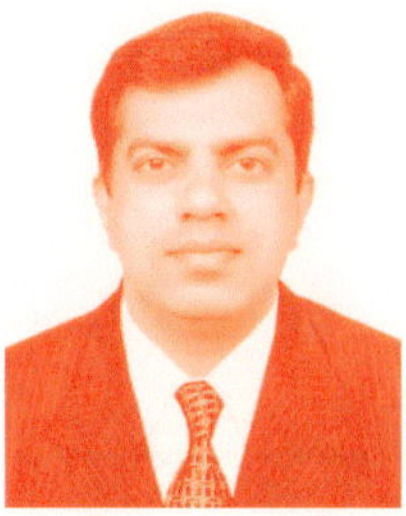
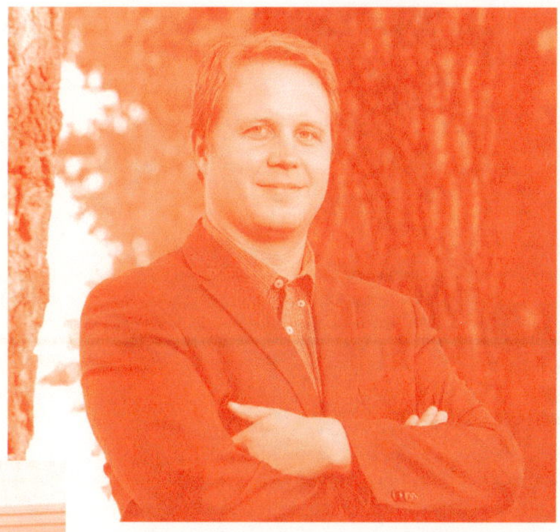
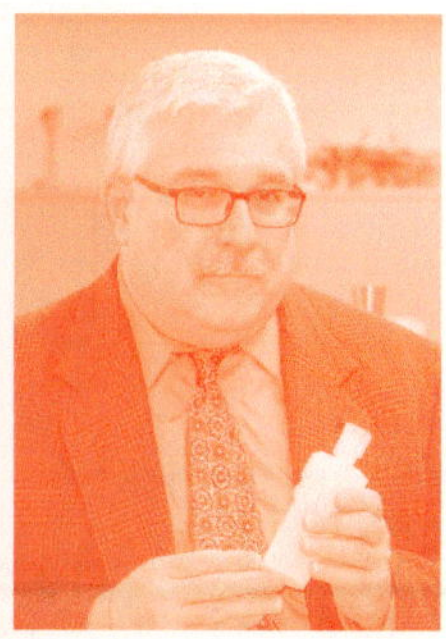
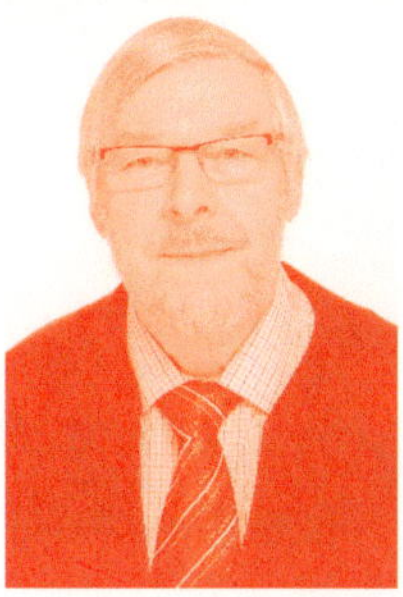
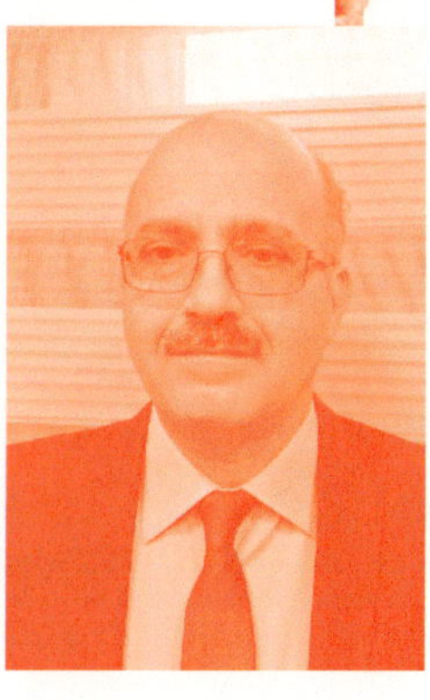
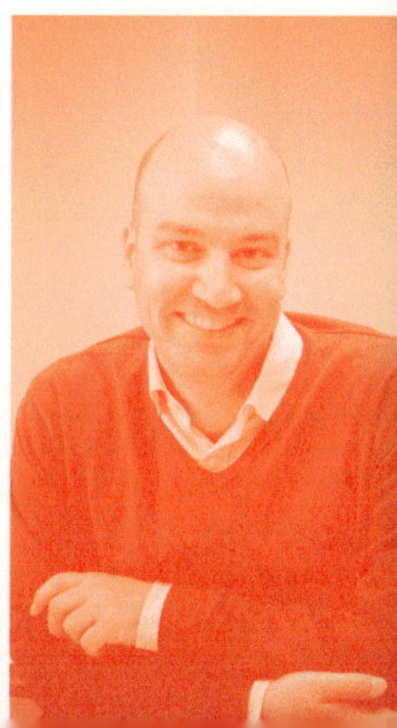
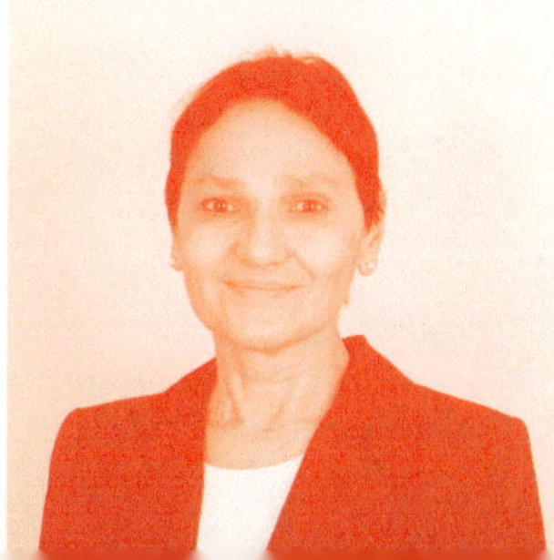

Urinary Tract Infection and Nephropathy - Insights into Potential Relationship
http://dx.doi.org/10.5772/intechopen.91541
Edited by Ran Pang

Contributors
Jean Jeanov Filipov, Emil Paskalev Dimitrov, Muhamed Ali Al Kabe, Eman Th. Nadhaif Al-Fatlawy, Shiela Chetri, Akosua Bonsu Karikari, Courage Kosi Setsoafia Saba, David Yembilla Yamik, Hussein O. M. Al-Dahmoshi, Noor S.K Salman Al-Khafaji, Farah T. Al-Alaq, Elfiani Elfiani, Huntari Harahap, Omar Sherin Ragy, Patrick Hamilton, Durga Kanigicherla, Rama Garg, Ran Pang

First published in London, United Kingdom, 2022 by IntechOpen
IntechOpen is the global imprint of INTECHOPEN LIMITED, registered in England and Wales, registration number: 11086078, 5 Princes Gate Court, London, SW7 2QJ, United Kingdom
Printed in Croatia

British Library Cataloguing-in-Publication Data
A catalogue record for this book is available from the British Library

Additional hard and PDF copies can be obtained from orders@intechopen.com

Urinary Tract Infection and Nephropathy - Insights into Potential Relationship
Edited by Ran Pang
p. cm.
Print ISBN 978-1-83968-683-2
Online ISBN 978-1-83968-684-9
eBook (PDF) ISBN 978-1-83968-685-6

For EU product safety concerns:
IN TECH d.o.o., Prolaz Marije Krucifikse Kozulić 3, 51000 Rijeka, Croatia, info@intechopen.com or visit our website at intechopen.com.

Meet the editor

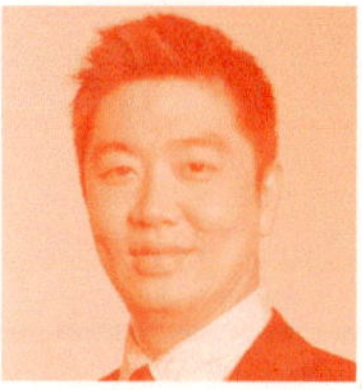

Ran Pang is a consultant urologist and a lead clinician in functional urology and urodynamics at Guang'anmen hospital, China Academy of Chinese Medical Sciences. After completing residency training, he was accepted to a clinical fellowship with Peking University in 2005. Subsequently, he joined a research fellowship at Mayo Clinic, USA in 2011, and a urodynamic fellowship at Dalhousie University, Canada in 2015. As a leading expert, Prof. Pang also serves on several international organizations as well as local professional committees. He is chair of the Publication and Communication Committee, International Continence Society, and vice-chair of the Pelvic Floor Disorder Group, Urology Committee, Chinese Association of Integrative Medicine. Additionally, he won the Albert Nelson Lifetime Achievement award in 2017.

Contents

Preface **XI**

Section 1
Introduction **1**

Chapter 1 **3**
Introductory Chapter: Insights into Urinary Disorders
by Ran Pang

Section 2
Insight into Kidney Diseases **9**

Chapter 2 **11**
Unraveling Primary Membranous Nephropathy Using Proteogenomic Studies
by Omar Ragy, Patrick Hamilton and Durga Kanigicherla

Chapter 3 **25**
Influence Engulfment Cell Motility-1 (ELMO-1) Protein and Matrix Metalloproteases-9 (MMP-9) in Diabetic Nephropathy Patients
by Elfiani Elfiani and Huntari Harahap

Chapter 4 **33**
Therapeutic Apheresis in Renal Transplantation: Indications and Strategies
by Jean Jeanov Filipov and Emil Paskalev Dimitrov

Section 3
New Features of the Host-Pathogen Relationship **49**

Chapter 5 **51**
Bacterial Resistance in Urinary Tract Infections: Multidrug Resistant ESBL Producing Gram Negative Uropathogens from Patients
by Akosua Bonsu Karikari, Courage Kosi Setsoafia Saba and David Yembilla Yamik

Chapter 6 **63**
Post-Covid-19 Era: What is Next?
by Shiela Chetri

Chapter 7 71
Virulence and Antibiotic Resistance of *Acinetobacter baumannii* among Urinary Tract Infections
by Hussein O.M. Al-Dahmoshi, Noor S.K. Al-Khafaji and Farah T. Al-Alaq

Chapter 8 87
Breakthrough Host Defense: UTI in Pregnant Women in Comparsion to Non-Pregnant
by Muhamed Ali Al Kabe and Eman Th. Nadhaif Al-Fatlawy

Chapter 9 97
Ureteric Injury in Gynecology Surgery
by Rama Garg

Preface

The kidneys, ureters, bladder, and urethra play an important role not only in urine production and transport but also in preventing the invasion of pathogens. In this book, experts from different countries demonstrate clinical and research advances in nephropathy and urinary tract infection.

Membranous nephropathy is a kind of antibody-mediated autoimmune glomerular disease. In their chapter, Dr. Omar Ragy et al. present the gene polymorphism in patients with membranous nephropathy, as well as discuss the value of proteomics and transcriptomic analysis in managing the disease. These modern techniques of analysis make it possible to minimize patients' immunosuppression exposure and identify the most effective targeted immunosuppressive therapy for each patient.

Diabetic nephropathy is a common cause of end-stage kidney disease. Interestingly, not all patients with diabetes mellitus will develop diabetic nephropathy. In their chapter, Drs. Elfiani Elfiani and Huntari Harahap present a cross-sectional comparative study to identify potential biomarkers for the occurrence of diabetic nephropathy.

A kidney transplant is considered the best treatment for patients with end-stage kidney disease. However, some conditions, such as antibody-mediated rejection and recurrent focal segmental glomerulosclerosis, may result in graft failure. Therapeutic apheresis is believed to be an effective treatment for managing these conditions since it can remove donor-specific antibodies and other circulating factors. In their chapter, Drs. Jean Jeanov Filipov and Emil Paskalev Dimitrov demonstrate the current evidence on the application of therapeutic apheresis.

Apart from urine transport, storage, and elimination, the urinary tract also acts as a barrier preventing pathogens from invading. Once pathogens break through the barrier, people will suffer from urinary tract infections. Due to the wide use of antibiotics, some bacteria have developed resistance to these drugs. In their chapter, Dr. Akosua Bonsu Karikari et al. present the characteristics of multidrug-resistant organisms isolated from patients with urinary tract infections in Northern Ghana.

Escherichia coli is the common pathogen causing urinary tract infection. Multidrug-resistant Escherichia coli has attracted broad attention. Dr. Shiela Chetri points out multidrug efflux pumps encoded in the microorganism's chromosomes are the main antibiotic-resistant mechanism in *E. coli*.

Acinetobacter baumannii is a kind of opportunistic bacteria related to hospital-acquired infection. In their chapter, Dr. Hussein O.M. Al-Dahmoshi et al. reveal the virulence factors of *A. baumannii* resulting in urinary tract infection. This information allows clinicians to develop targeted treatment strategies.

Besides the evolution of bacterial virulence, some conditions can also cause the body to be susceptible to urinary tract infection. Of those, pregnancy is one of the most common since it may result in temporary ureteral dilation and hydronephrosis. In their chapter, Drs. Muhamed Ali Al Kabe and Eman Th. Nadhaif Al-Fatlawy perform a case-control study that shows pregnant women are at significantly increased risk of bacteriuria.

An intact urothelium and a normal anatomical structure of the urinary tract are the foundation of a powerful barrier. Iatrogenic injury is a common factor that impairs epithelial integrity and consequently weakens the function of the barrier. In general, ureteric injuries in gynecology surgery are one of the most common Iatrogenic injuries of the urinary tract. Dr. Rama Garg presents the diagnosis, treatment, and prevention of ureteric injury in gynecology surgery.

Although this book does not cover all aspects of urinary tract infection and nephropathy, it provides readers with important updates.

Ran Pang
Department of Urology,
Guang'anmen Hospital,
China Academy of Chinese Medical Sciences,
Beijing, China

Section 1

Introduction

Chapter 1

Introductory Chapter: Insights into Urinary Disorders

Ran Pang

1. Introduction

Kidney, ureter, and bladder are the important urinary organs, which not only produce and transport urine, but also play a role as a barrier to prevent the invasion of pathogens [1]. Once any of them has dysfunction or damage, others can be affected. It has been a clinical issue how to prevent these organs from damage.

2. Insight into the dysfunction of kidney and bladder

The foundation protecting the function of these urinary organs is to understand their pathophysiology and risk prediction on a deeper level. Recently, the advances in genomics, proteomics, and metabolomics provide clinicians and researchers with the novel insights into this field.

Membranous nephropathy is one of the most common causes of adult nephrotic syndrome, which presents a significantly high risk to progress to end-stage kidney disease [2]. Its pathogenesis had been unknown until M-type phospholipase A2 receptor (PLA2R) was identified, which confirmed membranous nephropathy was a kind of antibody-mediated autoimmune glomerular disease [3]. Subsequently, thrombospondin type-1 domain-containing 7A (THSD7A) was found as another target antigen in patients with anti-PLA2R-negative membranous nephropathy [4]. Some studies revealed that the level of PLA2R was correlated with the activity of membranous nephropathy and the effectiveness of immunosuppression [5, 6]. Another study showed that the persistence of serum anti-THSD7A antibodies suggested a high recurrence risk of membranous nephropathy in the patients underwent renal transplant [7].

Diabetic nephropathy is another common cause for patients to suffer end-stage kidney disease. Interestingly, not all the patients with diabetes mellitus will eventually develop into diabetic nephropathy. It has been revealed that genetic susceptibility plays a role in pathogenesis of diabetic nephropathy [8]. A number of studies demonstrated some genes including ELMO1, APOC1, ACE, AKR1B1, APOE, CHN2, EPO, GREM1, NOS3, HSPG2, FRMD3, CPVL, VEGFA, CARS, and UNC13B were associated with diabetic nephropathy [9, 10]. Of those, ELMO1 is the most prevalent one associated with diabetic nephropathy risk, which is located on chromosome 7 p14.1–2. The result from a meta-analysis showed the relationship between ELMO1 and diabetic nephropathy exclusively in Asia population with diabetes mellitus [11]. Traditionally, microalbuminuria has been considered as the main standard for early diagnosis of diabetic nephropathy. However, its predictive value for diabetic nephropathy is being questioned because a number of conditions, including hyperglycemia, hypertension, infections, stress, severe sports and cardiovascular decompensation, may contribute to the false-positive result [12]. Furthermore, microalbuminuria cannot detect the early stage of diabetic nephropathy since its appearance is generally secondary to the glomerular damage [13]. Proteomics provides an insight into the risk prediction of early diabetic nephropathy and prevention of late-stage kidney damage, because not only the structure and function of a series of proteins are analyzed, but also the interaction among proteins is measured. Based on the proteome analysis, several proteins present the predictive value for kidney damage in patients with diabetic nephropathy. Basically, these proteins can be classified into three groups. Vitamin D-binding protein (VDBP) and neutrophil gelatinase-associated lipocalin (NGAL) are considered as the biomarkers related to tubular damage in patients with diabetic nephropathy. The elevated levels of those proteins in either serum or urine normally indicate potential renal tubular dysfunction [14]. It has been reported that GPC5, ANGPTL4, and soluble Klotho could be the biomarkers detecting glomerular damage [14]. Additionally, MCP-1, as an inflammation-related biomarker, has been used to predict the development of diabetic nephropathy [14].

Besides kidney diseases, interstitial cystitis/bladder pain syndrome (IC/BPS) is a common bladder storage dysfunction, which causes patients severe storage lower urinary tract symptoms (LUTS). Currently, the exact etiology of IC/BPS is still not fully understood and no gold standard is available for the diagnosis of IC/BPS. With the development of proteomics and metabolomics, a set of urine biomarkers associated with IC/BPS were found, which allows clinicians to understand IC/BPS at the molecular level. Tonyali et al. found that IC/BPS patients presented a significantly higher level in urinary nerve growth factor (NGF) normalized to urine creatinine compared with healthy controls [15]. Macrophage inhibitory factor (MIF) is another potential biomarker, which was found to be significantly increased in IC/BPS patients in comparison with control groups. Its reported sensitivity, specificity, and AUC in detecting IC/BPS were 47%, 91% and 0.730, respectively, using MIF normalized to urine creatinine [16]. In addition, Parker et al. [17] identified six metabolites associated with IC/BPS using liquid chromatography-high-resolution mass spectrometric. Of those, etiocholan-3alpha-ol-17-one (Etio-S) was considered as a good predictor for IC/BPS, with a sensitivity of 91.2%, a specificity of 87.4%, and AUC of 0.92.

3. A powerful barrier to pathogen invasion

Apart from urine transport, storage, and elimination, kidney, ureter and bladder also act as a barrier preventing pathogens from invading. On one hand, intact urothelium and normal anatomical structure and function of urinary tract are the foundation of a powerful barrier. Any anatomical or physiological abnormality related to urinary system may weaken the barrier, which makes the body vulnerable to pathogens. On the other hand, evolution of bacterial virulence and acquisition of antibiotic resistance make the pathogens more invasive. Once the host defense is not strong enough to resist microbial attack, the body will suffer from urinary tract infection (UTI).

Bladder outlet obstruction is one of the most common anatomic abnormalities of lower urinary tract, which significantly increases UTI risk [18]. In general, the causes of bladder outlet obstruction include urethral stricture, bladder neck obstruction, and, in men, benign prostatic hyperplasia. Of those, benign prostatic hyperplasia is the most common reason in the aging male population. It is reported that the prevalence of bacteriuria in men with benign prostatic hyperplasia ranges from 4.4 to 44.7% [19]. According to some guidelines, recurrent or persistent UTI is considered as an indication for surgical treatment in men with benign prostatic hyperplasia [18, 20].

Vesicoureteral reflux (VUR) is a common congenital anatomic abnormality in children, which is closely associated with high risk of UTI. The prevalence of VUR is approximately 1% in general population and is significantly increased in children [21, 22]. It is reported that 30 ~ 40% of children with VUR experience recurrent UTI [23]. VUR is graded from I (mild) to V (severe) based on the height of reflux up the ureter and degree of dilatation of the ureter. The higher grade the VUR is, the higher risk the patients develop renal failure in future due to the renal scars secondary to UTI. Therefore, it is important to prevent and manage UTI in patients with VUR. Traditionally, antibiotic prophylaxis has been considered as an effective strategy to prevent UTI in patients with VUR. However, a meta-analysis including four randomized controlled trials (RCTs) did not demonstrate a clear benefit of antibiotic prophylaxis in children with grades I and II VUR [24]. Although a later meta-analysis including eight RCTs showed the effectiveness of antibiotic prophylaxis in preventing recurrent UTI, the majority of the studies were at high risk of bias, which significantly weaken the certainty of evidence [25]. Surgical correction is a therapeutic strategy for high grade of VUR with a successful rate of 80 ~ 93% [26, 27].

Besides anatomic defects, the physiological abnormalities resulting from a series of conditions, such as pregnancy, diabetes mellitus, and renal failure, can also cause the body to be susceptible to UTI. Of those, pregnancy is the most common reason resulting in the temporary physiological abnormalities in women. On one hand, the enlarged uterus during pregnancy may compress the bladder and ureter, causing ureteral dilation and hydronephrosis. On the other hand, the changes in hormone levels stemming from the pregnancy can induce the relaxation of ureteric smooth muscles, which contributes to the urine retention in the renal-collecting system and ureter. As a result, the dilated renal pelvic and ureter provide a permissive environment for pathogens to grow and reproduce. In general, the prevention of UTI in these cases should be based on the management of the coexisted conditions.

With the broad-spectrum antibiotics being widely used, the bacteria continue to evolve *via* developing various defense mechanisms. In general, bacterial pathogens can achieve drug resistance through three different biochemical pathways [28]. Firstly, bacteria can mutate genes encoding the target site of antibiotics and consequently survive in the presence of the antimicrobial molecule. Secondary, bacteria can upregulate the expression of efflux pumps, which result in antibiotic resistance due to extruding the drug out of the cell. Finally, bacteria can produce some special proteins that interfere with the target site the antibiotics act on. In terms of specific bacteria, *Escherichia coli* producing extended spectrum beta-lactamases (ESBL) is the most common drug-resistant pathogen causing refractory UTI. Although there are no specific data regarding the prevalence of ESBL-positive *E. coli* in UTI, the percentage of ESBL-positive *E. coli* isolated from bloodstream showed a significantly increase over the past years [29]. The management for UTI caused by ESBL-positive *E. coli* remains a challenge since the majority of antibiotics have no effect on the drug-resistant pathogen. Based on current evidence, fosfomycin trometamol appears to be a therapeutic option because of its broad spectrum of activity against both Gram-negative bacteria.

4. Summary

With the development in genomics, proteomics, and metabolomics, a series of findings bring some novel insights into the pathophysiology and potential etiology of urinary tract disorders, which allows clinicians to perform personalized treatment for patients. Besides, a number of recent studies, which reveal host susceptibility factors and changes in bacterial virulence, provide important information for clinicians in making prevention strategies for UTI.

Author details

Ran Pang
Guang'anmen Hospital, China Academy of Chinese Medical Sciences,
Beijing, China

*Address all correspondence to: pangran2002@gmail.com

References

[1] Apodaca G. The uroepithelium: Not just a passive barrier. Traffic. 2004;**5**(3): 117-128

[2] Go AS, Tan TC, Chertow GM, Ordonez JD, Fan D, Law D, et al. Primary nephrotic syndrome and risks of ESKD, cardiovascular events, and death: The kaiser permanente nephrotic syndrome study. J Am Soc Nephrol. 2021;**32**(9):2303-2314

[3] Beck LH Jr, Bonegio RG, Lambeau G, Beck DM, Powell DW, Cummins TD, et al. M-type phospholipase A2 receptor as target antigen in idiopathic membranous nephropathy. The New England Journal of Medicine. 2009;**361**(1):11-21

[4] Tomas NM, Beck LH Jr, Meyer-Schwesinger C, Seitz-Polski B, Ma H, Zahner G, et al. Thrombospondin type-1 domain-containing 7A in idiopathic membranous nephropathy. The New England Journal of Medicine. 2014;**371**(24):2277-2287

[5] Bomback AS. Management of membranous nephropathy in the PLA2R era. Clinical Journal of the American Society of Nephrology. 2018;**13**(5): 784-786

[6] Hoxha E, Thiele I, Zahner G, Panzer U, Harendza S, Stahl RA. Phospholipase A2 receptor autoantibodies and clinical outcome in patients with primary membranous nephropathy. J Am Soc Nephrol. 2014;**25**(6):1357-1366

[7] Tomas NM, Hoxha E, Reinicke AT, Fester L, Helmchen U, Gerth J, et al. Autoantibodies against thrombospondin type 1 domain-containing 7A induce membranous nephropathy. The Journal of Clinical Investigation. 2016;**126**(7):2519-2532

[8] Mambiya M, Shang M, Wang Y, Li Q, Liu S, Yang L, et al. The play of genes and non-genetic factors on type 2 diabetes. Frontiers in Public Health. 2019;**7**:349

[9] Reddy BM, Pranavchand R, Latheef SAA. Overview of genomics and post-genomics research on type 2 diabetes mellitus: Future perspectives and a framework for further studies. Journal of Biosciences. 2019;**44**(1):21

[10] Regine I, Husain R, Aswathi RP, Reddy DR, Ahmed S, Ramakrishnan V. Association between PPARγrs1801282 polymorphism with diabetic nephropathy and type-2 diabetes mellitus susceptibility in south India and a meta-analysis. Nefrología. 2020;**40**(3):287-298

[11] Mooyaart AL, Valk EJ, van Es LA, Bruijn JA, de Heer E, Freedman BI, et al. Genetic associations in diabetic nephropathy: A meta-analysis. Diabetologia. 2011;**54**(3):544-553

[12] Sims EK, Evans-Molina C. Urinary biomarkers for the early diagnosis of retinopathy and nephropathy in type 1 diabetes mellitus: A "steady stream" of information using proteomics. Translational Research: The Journal of Laboratory and Clinical Medicine. 2014;**163**(3):183-187

[13] Elsheikh M, Elhefnawy KA, Emad G, Ismail M, Borai M. Zinc alpha 2 glycoprotein as an early biomarker of diabetic nephropathy in patients with type 2 diabetes mellitus. Jornal Brasileiro de Nefrologia: 'Orgao Oficial de Sociedades Brasileira e Latino-Americana de Nefrologia. 2019;**41**(4): 509-517

[14] Sauriasari R, Safitri DD, Azmi NU. Current updates on protein as biomarkers for diabetic kidney disease: A systematic review. Therapeutic Advances in Endocrinology and Metabolism. 2021;**12**:20420188211049612

[15] Tonyali S, Ates D, Akbiyik F, Kankaya D, Baydar D, Ergen A. Urine nerve growth factor (NGF) level, bladder nerve staining and symptom/problem scores in patients with interstitial cystitis. Advances in Clinical and Experimental Medicine: Official Organ Wroclaw Medical University. 2018;**27**(2):159-163

[16] Vera PL, Preston DM, Moldwin RM, Erickson DR, Mowlazadeh B, Ma F, et al. Elevated urine levels of macrophage migration inhibitory factor in inflammatory bladder conditions: A potential biomarker for a subgroup of interstitial cystitis/bladder pain syndrome patients. Urology. 2018;**116**:55-62

[17] Parker KS, Crowley JR, Stephens-Shields AJ, van Bokhoven A, Lucia MS, Lai HH, et al. Urinary metabolomics identifies a molecular correlate of interstitial cystitis/bladder pain syndrome in a multidisciplinary approach to the study of chronic pelvic pain (MAPP) research network cohort. eBioMedicine. 2016;7:167-174

[18] Sabih A, Leslie SW. Complicated Urinary Tract Infections. Treasure Island (FL). Copyright © 2021: StatPearls Publishing LLC; 2021

[19] Agbugui JO, Obarisiagbon EO, Osaigbovo II. Bacteriology of urine specimens obtained from men with symptomatic benign prostatic hyperplasia. Nigerian Journal of Surgery: Official Publication of the Nigerian Surgical Research Society. 2016;**22**(2):65-69

[20] Homma Y, Gotoh M, Kawauchi A, Kojima Y, Masumori N, Nagai A, et al. Clinical guidelines for male lower urinary tract symptoms and benign prostatic hyperplasia. International Journal of Urology: Official Journal of the Japanese Urological Association. 2017;**24**(10):716-729

[21] Chapman CJ, Bailey RR, Janus ED, Abbott GD, Lynn KL. Vesicoureteric reflux: Segregation analysis. American Journal of Medical Genetics. 1985;**20**(4): 577-584

[22] Garin EH. Primary vesicoureteral reflux; what have we learnt from the recently published randomized, controlled trials? Pediatric Nephrology (Berlin, Germany). 2019;**34**(9): 1513-1519

[23] Mårild S, Jodal U. Incidence rate of first-time symptomatic urinary tract infection in children under 6 years of age. Acta Paediatrica (Oslo, Norway: 1992). 1998;**87**(5):549-552

[24] Montini G, Hewitt I. Urinary tract infections: To prophylaxis or not to prophylaxis? Pediatric nephrology (Berlin, Germany). 2009;**24**(9): 1605-1609

[25] Wang HH, Gbadegesin RA, Foreman JW, Nagaraj SK, Wigfall DR, Wiener JS, et al. Efficacy of antibiotic prophylaxis in children with vesicoureteral reflux: Systematic review and meta-analysis. The Journal of Urology. 2015;**193**(3):963-969

[26] Akhavan A, Avery D, Lendvay TS. Robot-assisted extravesical ureteral reimplantation: Outcomes and conclusions from 78 ureters. Journal of Pediatric Urology. 2014;**10**(5):864-868

[27] Arlen AM, Broderick KM, Travers C, Smith EA, Elmore JM, Kirsch AJ. Outcomes of complex robot-assisted extravesical ureteral reimplantation in the pediatric population. Journal of Pediatric Urology. 2016;**12**(3):169.e1-169.e6

[28] Munita JM, Arias CA. Mechanisms of antibiotic resistance. Microbiology Spectrum. 2016;**4**(2):1-37

[29] Mazzariol A, Bazaj A, Cornaglia G. Multi-drug-resistant Gram-negative bacteria causing urinary tract infections: A review. Journal of Chemotherapy (Florence, Italy). 2017;**29**(Suppl. 1):2-9

Section 2

Insight into Kidney Diseases

Chapter 2

Unraveling Primary Membranous Nephropathy Using Proteogenomic Studies

Omar Ragy, Patrick Hamilton and Durga Kanigicherla

Abstract

Membranous nephropathy is one of the leading causes of nephrotic syndrome in adults. The disease manifests in different forms with varying severity and outcomes range from spontaneous remission to rapid disease progression. The effects of the disease are so far best understood using conventional histopathological morphology and clinical phenotype. Being an autoimmune condition subject to a multi-hit hypothesis, the notion of underlying genetic risks is being examined in recent times. Current evidence points to significant heterogeneity in the gene expression profiles in both the immune system and at the glomerular level, with potential implications for disease management. Further proteomic and transcriptomic analysis can instruct classification, prognostication, and treatment pathways. This chapter focuses on the links identified between primary membranous nephropathy and underlying gene polymorphism, and pathways using both proteomics and transcriptomic analysis. We discuss the potential impact this could have on future management to try to minimize the patient's immunosuppression exposure and find the most effective targeted immunosuppressive therapy.

Keywords: membranous nephropathy, gene polymorphism, HLA, Transcriptomics, Proteomics

1. Introduction

Management of membranous nephropathy remains a continuing challenge in the field of nephrology. Over the last 50 years, we have been classifying and managing membranous nephropathy based on both histological and clinical phenotyping, which is the key feature guiding treatment decisions. However, in recent years other mechanisms have come to shed light on the heterogeneity of membranous nephropathy and clinical outcomes. With the emergence of proteogenomic analysis, the classification of other nephrotic syndromes has advanced immensely [1]. Therefore, the potential value for membranous nephropathy is to be considered.

Varied clinical manifestation may be due to the polymorphic gene expression in the immune system as well as at the glomerular filtration barrier site, which comprises podocytes, endothelial cells, and intervening glomerular basement membrane [2]. In addition to the multiple immune cascade pathways, underlying complex molecular and cellular processes are identified by proteomics and transcriptomics in glomerular disorders like Minimal Change Disease and focal segmental glomerulosclerosis (FSGS) [1]. Early data suggest that gene expression and molecular pathways are both potential emerging therapeutic targets in the era of precision medicine in these disorders.

Primary membranous nephropathy is considered an autoimmune disease, associated with autoantibodies recognizing a target antigen on the podocytes. The connection between the immune system and underlying cellular pathways in the pathophysiology of membranous nephropathy has been an area of extensive research. Even though membranous nephropathy does not follow the mendelian trait, the role of underlying genetic factors was examined in previous studies.

Although clinical and histological apparency of membranous nephropathy are seemingly similar, response to immunosuppressive therapy can be variable with poor response to treatment in some patients whilst about a third of the patients have minimal to no long-term consequence following spontaneous remission. This heterogenicity may be due to differences in underlying biological processes influenced by genetic polymorphism and protein interaction networks and this warrants more in-depth understanding to unravel precise prognostication and therapeutic options.

The genome-wide association study (GWAS) provided evidence on the susceptibility of specific HLA regions and the susceptibility to primary membranous nephropathy [3]. With the emergence of PLA_2R antigen as an immune system target in primary membranous nephropathy, more evidence has shown a link between PLA_2R antigen and specific HLA alleles [4, 5].

This chapter intends to review the current understanding of gene expression analysis, proteomics, and metabolomics in membranous nephropathy with a focus on the utility of these methods in clinical practice.

2. Integrating genomics, transcriptomics, and proteomics

The major histocompatibility complex found on chromosome 6 p21 consists of polymorphic genes that code cell surface proteins and plays an important role in adaptive immunity. MHC I is found on all nucleated cells whereas MHC II is found mainly on antigen-presenting cells. The human genome project has been a turning point in our understanding of human genomes and our understanding of disease pathophysiology [6], revealing the link between genetic downstream pathways for both target antigens and immune cells.

It has been found that immune-mediated glomerular injury involves activation of both innate and adaptive immunity, which leads to the clinical and pathological manifestation of the disease. Over the past 10 years, more than 80 genes causing glomerular barrier dysfunction have been identified [2]. With the emergence of human genetic studies, understanding which gene sequence is the main trigger for the immune system malfunction became a very powerful tool to uncover the molecular drivers of these diseases and help find potential targeted therapy.

The understanding of genome sequence will reveal the gene expression and how the cell behaves in a static state by looking at the amino acid sequence of the DNA. To identify the effect of variation in genetic architecture on proteins and correlate with diseases, one needs to move to undertake transcriptomics and proteomics, to study mRNA from DNA code and tRNA decoding the mRNA sequence into protein. This function can further vary by an alternative splicing process where the single genome can be translated into different proteins [7]. Hence, this is a process that captures the expressed portion of the genome and the expressed protein set in the genome, which will reveal how the cells act in a dynamic state as well as a static state [8].

Proteomic analysis is performed directly from tissue microdissection and mass spectrometry. The NEPTUNE group identified clusters of patients based on their mRNA expression in the tubulointerstitial portion of renal tissue [1]. Also, they performed non-invasive techniques to evaluate the proteomic biomarkers and found common downstream gene expression pathways from the one found in the renal tissues. The utility of proteomics in autoimmune kidney diseases has been previously tested and has shown common cellular pathways that might help in targeting therapy for different autoimmune renal conditions [9, 10].

Membranous nephropathy is one of the leading causes of nephrotic syndromes. At the histological level, both glomerular immunoglobulin and complement deposition are hallmarks in making the diagnosis. PLA_2R1 antigen was the first membrane-bound glycoprotein identified as a target antigen in adults with primary membranous nephropathy. This was identified by Beck *et al* in a pivotal study in 2009. With the use of laser microdissection and mass spectrometry LM/MS, new target antigens are being discovered, some of which may present opportunities to identify as protein biomarkers for secondary autoimmune or malignancy-associated membranous nephropathy [11, 12]. The absence of PLA_2R antigen on histological staining and the presence of Exostosin1/2 identified on mass spectrometry following laser microdissection can pave the way for identifying Lupus class 5 at an early stage [13]. Also identifying NELL1 by laser microdissection and mass spectrometry can allow early evaluation for underlying malignancy and may warrant further follow-up [14]. Validation of these target antigens in independent studies will add further value to the clinical management of these patients.

Another attractive area for the use of laser microdissection and mass spectrometry is Amyloidosis. Due to the abundance of amyloid protein in the tissue, LM/MS has gained investigators' attention and showed very encouraging outcomes when performed on amyloid renal tissue samples [15].

Even though both transcriptomics and proteomics yield very rich information, they have some limitations. This may be due to the alterations that might happen after mRNA translation or failure to identify proteins resulting from the alternative splicing process. Yet, these are complementary information and one can still conclude within these limitations [16].

3. Role of immunoglobulins in the disease pathophysiology

During the early development of T and B cells as the immune system line of defense, a VDJ (variable diversity joining) gene segment is created. Due to the heterogeneous gene sequence resulting from mutation triggers, diverse antibodies and T cell receptors are formed given the variable amino acid sequence identified on these cell's genes [17]. IgG3 is the least VDJ mutated followed by IgG1, IgG2 then IgG4. Based on this finding, a temporal model for immunoglobulin subclass transformation during an inflammatory response has been hypothesized [18]. This suggests that cells first switch from IgM to IgG3, to IgG1, to IgG2 finally to IgG4 following a genomic ordering. That was partially similar to the Markov chain except for IgG2 emerging before IgG1 [19]. IgG1 is a complement-fixing antibody with IgG4 lacking the effector response of antibody-dependent cell-mediated cytotoxicity and complement-dependent cellular toxicity but is known for its anti-inflammatory blocking response, which can dampen down the overactivity of other IgG subclasses [20].

The role of immunoglobulin subtypes and their effect on complement when identified by immunofluorescent stain on renal tissue of membranous nephropathy is an area that requires further research. In one study, there has been a correlation between serum IgG4 and PLA2R associated membranous nephropathy disease activity [21]. Subclassing the immunoglobulin types can also be performed using laser microdissection and mass spectrometry at the tissue level. It has been found that IgG1 is the most abundant subclass followed by IgG4 in Exostosin1/2 associated membranous nephropathy compared to IgG4 in PLA_2R associated membranous nephropathy [11]. This is in line with other studies [19, 22]. This raises the question if the response to immunosuppression varies based on these antibodies' amino acid sequence or not. Same for the downstream cellular and molecular pathways resulting from the inflammatory cascade rather than relying on the immunoglobulin subtype staining.

4. Role of complements in the disease pathophysiology

Identifying complements on routine renal biopsy evaluation gives us a limited understanding of the role of these complements in the disease process. Complement proteins and their cleavage products have a vital role in attacking the glomerular basement membrane and podocytes [23]. Yet, most of the randomized controlled trials were designed to use immunosuppression medication directed towards blocking the immune system at the immunoglobulin level rather than targeting complements and the underlying cellular and molecular pathways identified by proteogenomic analysis [24–27] (RI-CYCLO NCT03018535).

Although the 3 complement pathways (classical, lectin, and alternative) converge at the same downstream target, they differ from each other at the point of origin [23]. The classical pathway is mainly triggered by IgM and IgG3/1 complexing with the antigen. This immune complex activates C1, which is the main classical complement pathway protein. The C1 complex then breaks down C2 and C4 into C2b and C4a, which then merge to form the C3 convertase. The lectin pathway is activated when the mannose-binding lectin attaches to the bacterial surface. This complex further aids the classical pathway by the breakdown of C2 and C4 and leads to the formation of C3 convertase. The alternative pathway is activated by the spontaneous hydrolysis of C3 into C3b, which binds to factor B and forms the other C3 convertase. This pathway abrogation is being investigated in the ongoing clinical trial utilizing LNP023 (NCT04154787). Finally, c3 convertase from classical, lectin, and alternative pathway complexes with c3b to form two different types of c5 convertase that cascades to form the membrane attack complex as the final complement effector.

Eculizumab is a humanized monoclonal antibody that inhibits the cleavage of C5 into C5a and C5b and hence inhibits the deployment of membrane attach complex. In 2002, an abstract of a randomized control trial in 200 patients with idiopathic membranous nephropathy received 2 dose regimens of eculizumab with no significant effect on neither proteinuria nor renal function [28]. This was probably due to an inadequate complement inhibition response and further trials with higher doses may be required.

The role of complement activation in membranous nephropathy glomerular injury is supported by the presence of C3, C5b-9, and IgG in the subepithelial space. With the discovery of IgG4 as the main subclass antibody identified in primary membranous nephropathy, it should be noted that these antibodies are incapable of binding to C1q and therefore unable to activate the classical complement pathway and are unlikely to be present in primary membranous nephropathy. The absence of C1q in the presence of C4d which is a classical pathway protein break down from C4b has been identified in cases of primary membranous nephropathy. The most likely explanation is that either there is an element of classical pathway activation that has not been discovered yet, or the lectin pathway has been activated. Lectin pathway activation has shown to carry a worse prognosis in PLA_2R associated membranous nephropathy [29].

With the emergence of proteogenomic analysis, recent evidence has shed the light on the significance of complement activation in the pathophysiology of membranous nephropathy [22]. To further analyze, common target antigens for both primary and secondary autoimmune membranous nephropathy were identified using mass spectrometry following laser microdissection. Using these methods, they found PLA_2R antigen and Exostosin1/2 were the two most common target antigens for primary and secondary autoimmune membranous nephropathy respectively and were analyzed accordingly [11].

It has been found that the three complement pathways play a role in disease pathogenesis. Regardless of the antigen identified, C3 and its regulatory protein CFH as the main alternative pathway downstream proteins showed the highest spectral counts, whereas C1q as the main classical pathway downstream protein showed the lowest spectral count [22]. Moreover, they found high spectral counts from the terminal complement pathway cascade (C5, C6, C7, C8, and C9). Thus, targeting the terminal complement pathway might be a future therapeutic option. On a further note, investigators identified C4 as the second most abundant protein in the absence of Manon-binding lectin serine protease 1 and 2, which points to the role of the classical pathway in the underlying disease process.

The mannose-binding lectin molecule is a major recognition molecule of the lectin pathway. Genetic polymorphism has been shown to play a role in the disease downstream pathways. By performing genotyping, one study has found that patients with MBL deficiency can develop membranous nephropathy with the downstream complements being activated primarily from the alternative pathway. Whereas patients with wild type of MBL2 have their complements mainly derived from the lectin pathway [30]. These studies show that classical, lectin, and alternative complement pathways play a significant role in disease pathogenesis.

As previously discussed, the lectin pathway plays an important role in disease pathogenesis [30]. In a case–control Brazilian study, an association was noted between membranous nephropathy and mannose-binding lectin 2(MBL2) polymorphism in patients carrying O allele, in particular, A/O genotype [31]. Investigators also found a defective MBL production in patients with YA/O, XA/O, and O/O genotypes. As shown previously, activating the lectin pathway in patients with PLA_2R associated membranous nephropathy carries a worse prognosis [29].

The use of LM/MS is not limited to identifying proteins but also can aid in classifying disease severity and treatment response by analyzing the complement protein spectral counts [22]. The persistence of complements on glomerular capillaries may explain the lag in clinical remission behind immunological remission and provide a reason for persistent proteinuria after the disappearance of PLA_2R-Ab in serum [32]. More studies using proteogenomic analysis can further analyze these complement proteins to identify a more targeted therapy and inform about disease severity and likely response.

5. Single nucleotide polymorphism and genotyping in HLA class II allele and PLA_2R1 antigen

The immune system recognizes peptide sequences processed from a target antigen when presented by the antigen-presenting cells. In PLA_2R associated membranous nephropathy, the immune system will interpret the PLA_2R1 presented by the HLA Class II molecule as the target antigen. The GWAS (genome-wide association studies) identified a strong association of single nucleotide polymorphisms (SNPs) on both HLA-DQA1, PLA_2R1 antigen, and Primary Membranous nephropathy [4]. Due to the proximity of HLA-DQ and HLA-DR on chromosome 6 and the probability of linkage disequilibrium that can result in the coinheritance of common haplotype, both alleles were found to be associated with membranous nephropathy. When imputation was performed it has confirmed the same signals on the same loci identified in other studies [33]. That can also be interpreted from one study where they have identified a significant association between PLA_2R1 antigen and both HLA DQA1/DRB1 [34]. In the former study, it was noted that using a combined genetic risk score and serum anti PLA_2R antibody using the ELISA method can potentially mitigate the need for a diagnostic renal biopsy in high-risk patients.

Not all cases of primary membranous nephropathy are associated with PLA_2R1 antigen. After the discovery of the PLA_2R antigen, THSD7A was the 2nd antigen implicated in primary membranous nephropathy and is found in 2–5% of patients [35]. Investigators have identified similarities and differences between THSD7A and PLA_2R antigens [36]. This can be extrapolated to suggest that there may be an HLA link with THSD7A either similar or different to PLA_2R antigen. In a large case–control study, the link between the HLA-DQA1 and PLA_2R1 antigen was found to be more prevalent in patients with confirmed PLA_2R1 associated membranous nephropathy compared to PLA_2R1 negative patients [37]. For now, the specific association is yet to be noted in anti-PLA_2R1 negative cases. Also, association with these SNPs is seen in patients with Caucasian backgrounds compared to patients from Afro-American origins.

Another Asian study found a strong association between HLADQA1 and PLA_2R1 antigen [38]. In this study investigators not only identified SNP variation on HLA-DQA1 but also found that AA and AG genotype carriers are at increased risk of developing primary membranous nephropathy compared to those carrying GG genotype. On the other hand, GG genotype on PLA_2R1 antigen SNP and AA genotype on another were encountered more frequently in subjects with primary membranous nephropathy. Two other Asian studies have identified other HLA risk alleles other than HLA-DQA1 in their cohorts of patients with primary membranous nephropathy [39, 40]. Again this raises the possibility of linkage disequilibrium.

Correlating the treatment response to the underlying genetic polymorphism is another area that is being investigated. A Chinese-Taiwanese study observed that haplotype H1 might carry a higher risk for disease progression when compared to H3 haplotype. The group found no relation between disease progression and underlying genetic polymorphism in PLA2rR1 antigen without the incidence of ESRD or death after therapy [41].

In another Spanish study, they found no association between survival and single nucleotide polymorphism in PLA_2R1 antigen. In the same study, AA and AG genotypes in HLA-DQA1 and AA genotype on PLA_2R1 antigen were shown to be associated with a trend towards immunosuppression treatment response compared to other genotypes [42]. Moreover, AA and AG genotypes on HLA-DQA1 SNP have shown significant protection for doubling of serum creatinine and progression to end-stage renal disease, without identifying any protective genotypes on PLA2R1 antigen.

A Chinese paper has highlighted the ethnic distribution difference in membranous nephropathy based on their HLA types [34]. They have found that DRB1*1501 is the major risk allele in the East Asian population, DQA1*0501 in Europeans, and DRB1*0301 in both ethnicities. This new finding can allow us to categorize high-risk patients from different background ethnicities based on their HLA type.

6. Genetic polymorphism other location than HLA alleles and PLA_2R1 antigens

In addition to the previously mentioned HLA alleles and PLA_2R1 polymorphism, many other genes were discovered to be linked with primary membranous nephropathy. It has been shown that TH2 cells are predominant in primary membranous nephropathy due to the presence of IgG4, which belongs to type 2 immune response [43]. TH2 cells are responsible for the secretion of IL4, IL 10, and TNF α as major cytokines. These cytokines can enhance the expression of the HLA molecule and lead to disease pathogenesis.

In a case–control study, TNFα and TNFd genotypes belonging to MHC class III were associated with primary membranous nephropathy [44]. It was noted in this study that for that association to occur, the underlying HLA was B8/DR3/DQ2. The influence of TNF α gene polymorphism on disease progression was not present for either of the TNF genotypes separately or in combination. The importance of TNF in clinical practice was examined in a small study of 10 patients who did not respond to maximum RAS blockade. Pentoxifylline is a phosphodiesterase inhibitor that is capable of lowering TNF α levels were used, and patients were followed up for 6 months. 9 out of 10 patients achieved remission with TNF α levels trending down in both plasma and urine [45].

Another study showed an association between specific IL4 and IL10 genotypes and membranous nephropathy [46]. This raises a particular question for future studies using interleukin inhibitors in membranous nephropathy.

7. Genetic polymorphism and the risk of cancer and thrombosis

Identifying PLA_2R antibodies has not yet changed our approach for excluding secondary causes for membranous nephropathy. KDIGO recommendations include performing a secondary work up to rule out autoimmune conditions, infections, and malignancies [47]. Recently with the use of laser microdissection and mass spectrometry, NELL1 antigen has shown an association with cancers [14]. Genotyping by Polymerase chain reaction has shown an association between specific gene polymorphism and cancers, and progression to end-stage renal disease. In one study investigators sub-classified patients with urokinase plasminogen activator polymorphism (Gene 3'-UTR) into groups based on their allele distribution either C/C or C/T. Although the number of patients was significantly higher in the CC group, patients with T/C genotype had a better trend towards renal survival and lower cancer incidence [48]. It should be noted that this gene polymorphism was not different from the control group.

A plasminogen activator inhibitor 1 gene polymorphism was examined to assess for correlation with disease activity, treatment response, and long-term prognosis [49]. Patients carrying 5G/5G genotype were more likely to attain complete remission, whereas 4G/4G and 4G/5G were more likely to develop renal disease progression, and 4G/4G showing no signs of remission. Patients carrying the 4G allele (4G/4G or 4G/5G) were more likely to develop coronary artery disease and peripheral vascular disease in comparison to carriers of the 5G allele, which was in line with another meta-analysis that showed a high risk of myocardial infarction in plasminogen activator inhibitor 1 4G/5G carriers [50]. It should be noted that in the former study, gene polymorphism was not different between membranous nephropathy patients and controls. Moreover, the number of patients carrying 4G allele was almost double that for 5G allele. These studies are single-center studies and need validation through well-designed multi-center trials to establish the relationship between polymorphism and disease outcomes. The framework of bio registries can help to validate the significance of these studies.

8. Genetic polymorphism on TLR, MYH9, NF-κB, and IRF4

The toll-like receptor expressed on the surface of the macrophage plays an important role in the link between innate immunity and adaptive immunity. TLR recognizes microbes leading to activation of downstream signals that result in the production of INF gamma. It is speculated that the association of TLR9 in membranous nephropathy might explain why and how infections can trigger the occurrence of membranous nephropathy. In a previous study, overexpression of TLR in the renal tissues was confirmed in lupus nephritis [51]. The same idea was tested in an Asian study to identify the link between TLR9 and the incidence of membranous nephropathy. Genotyping for TLR9 found a statistically significant difference between AA and GG genotypes on two specific SNPs loci on TLR9 when compared to controls [52]. Although the incidence of tubulointerstitial fibrosis was higher in the A-G haplotype when compared to the non-A-G haplotype, survival did not differ between the two groups. Another study investigated the association between membranous nephropathy and TLR4 specific gene polymorphism and found a statistically significant difference between A/G TLR4 genotype in membranous nephropathy and control, and no difference in haplotype frequency [53]. These observations suggest a possible association between membranous nephropathy and TLR4/9.

Myosin heavy chain 9 (MYH9) is expressed on most of the tissues that participate in the process of cell division and migration. Mutation in MYH9 was found to be associated with many renal diseases [54]. A difference in specific gene pleomorphism on MYH9 between membranous nephropathy and control was found [55]. On haplotype frequency, C-A was the common haplotype in membranous nephropathy and that was significantly different from controls.

NF-κB (nuclear factor kappa-light-chain-enhancer of activated B cells) is a complex protein that controls cytokine production and plays a key role in regulating the immune response to infection.

The most abundant SNP (rs230540) found on the NKFB1 locus was predicted to have a functional impact on specific immune cells. Investigators have found that the previously mentioned SNP locus is associated with higher mRNA expression of NFKB1 in whole blood [34, 56]. Coinciding with the NFKB1 pro-inflammatory effect, another UK study has found that membranous nephropathy risk haplotype at this same locus has shown a higher leucocyte signal [57]. Another SNP locus (rs9405192) on IRF4 has shown a major role in innate immunity activation. IRF4 IS A lymphocytic gene that regulates toll-like receptor activation signaling, which is under the control of NFKB1 complex [58]. This highlights that certain loci on NFKB1 and IRF4 play a crucial role in the underlying membranous nephropathy pathophysiology at the cellular pathway level.

9. Conclusion

The heterogenicity of clinical phenotypes and outcomes in membranous nephropathy could be related to the underlying complex molecular, cellular, and biological pathways. Both genomic and proteomic analysis are becoming widely available tools to interrogate these possibilities. Membranous nephropathy being an autoimmune condition, requires identification of potential antigenic peptides at the podocyte, glomerular capillaries, and basement membrane levels. The proteogenomic analysis will help reveal downstream pathways that arise from the interaction between these genes, which can occur either at the glomerular level or in the immune system pathway. Hence, understanding the pathophysiology and the close interaction between various arms of the immune system and ancillary pathways is crucial for future targeted therapy in membranous nephropathy.

Laser microdissection and mass spectrometry will likely be crucial in revealing the link between the antibody subtypes and newly discovered glomerular antigens, and the three different complement pathways. Even though the classical pathway does not play a major role, some evidence has shed the light on its involvement. Thus, further investigations into types of complement activation with targets at the molecular level should be an area for future research.

The advent of proteogenomic analysis has shown a link between HLA and PLA_2R antigen, but evidence for the link with THSD7A and other antigens is yet to be discovered. Also, the correlation between HLA and disease outcome is another area of interest that might further aid our future choice for immunosuppression treatment. A well-designed trial is required to correlate that link with disease outcome and treatment response.

Identifying certain high-risk alleles in patients with urokinase plasminogen activator gene polymorphism and plasminogen inhibitor activator 1 pleomorphism, has shown a probable association with cancers, thrombosis, disease progression, and remission response. This might pave the way for future discovery of certain genes that can identify cancer as a trigger for membranous nephropathy even if it would occur years after diagnosis. Also, can help with identifying patients who are more prone to venous thromboembolism and would benefit from anticoagulation. Moreover, patients who are more liable for disease progression can benefit from early immunosuppression treatment without the need for a period of watchful wait on RASS inhibition compared to other patients who might attain complete remission without the need for aggressive immunosuppression therapy.

Hence, the proteogenomic analysis is the way forward for identifying targeted immunosuppression therapy for membranous nephropathy in the era of precision medicine.

Author details

Omar Ragy*, Patrick Hamilton and Durga Kanigicherla
Manchester Royal infirmary, Manchester, UK

*Address all correspondence to: omarragy85@gmail.com

References

[1] Mariani L, Eddy S, Martini S, Eichinger F, Godfrey B, Nair V, et al. Redefining Nephrotic Syndrome in Molecular Terms: Outcome-associated molecular clusters and patient stratification with noninvasive surrogate biomarkers. bioRxiv. 2018;427880.

[2] Li AS, Ingham JF, Lennon R. Genetic Disorders of the Glomerular Filtration Barrier. Clin J Am Soc Nephrol. 2020;15(9):CJN.11440919.

[3] Mladkova N, Kiryluk K. Genetic complexities of the HLA region and idiopathic membranous nephropathy. J Am Soc Nephrol. 2017;28(5):1331-1334.

[4] Stanescu HC, Arcos-Burgos M, Medlar A, Bockenhauer D, Kottgen A, Dragomirescu L, et al. Risk HLA-DQA1 and PLA 2 R1 alleles in idiopathic membranous nephropathy . N Engl J Med. 2011;364(7):616-626.

[5] Le W, Shi J, Zhang T, Liu L, Qin H, Liang S. PLA2R-Related Membranous Nephropathy. J Am Soc Nephrol. 2017;28:1642-1650.

[6] Lander ES, Linton LM, Birren B, Nusbaum C, Zody MC, Baldwin J, et al. Erratum: Initial sequencing and analysis of the human genome: International human genome sequencing consortium (nature (2001) 409 (860-921)). Nature. 2001;412(6846):565-566.

[7] Nilsen TW, Graveley BR. Expansion of the eukaryotic proteome by alternative splicing. Nature. 2010;463(7280):457-463.

[8] Kumar D, Bansal G, Narang A, Basak T, Abbas T, Dash D. Integrating transcriptome and proteome profiling: Strategies and applications. Proteomics. 2016;16(19):2533-2544.

[9] Liu P, Lassén E, Nair V, Berthier CC, Suguro M, Sihlbom C, et al. Transcriptomic and proteomic profiling provides insight into mesangial cell function in IgA nephropathy. Vol. 28, Journal of the American Society of Nephrology. 2017. p. 2961-2972.

[10] Baker MA, Davis SJ, Liu P, Pan X, Williams AM, Iczkowski KA, et al. Tissue-specific MicroRNA expression patterns in four types of kidney disease. Vol. 28, Journal of the American Society of Nephrology. 2017. p. 2985-2992.

[11] Sethi S, Madden BJ, Debiec H, Cristine Charlesworth M, Gross L, Ravindran A, et al. Exostosin 1/ exostosin 2–associated membranous nephropathy. J Am Soc Nephrol. 2019;30(6):1123-1136.

[12] Sethi S, Debiec H, Madden B, Charlesworth MC, Morelle J, Gross LA, et al. Neural epidermal growth factor-like 1 protein (NELL-1) associated membranous nephropathy. Kidney Int [Internet]. 2020;97(1):163-174. Available from: https://doi.org/10.1016/j.kint.2019.09.014

[13] Ravindran A, Casal Moura M, Fervenza F, Nasr S, Alexander M, Fidler M et al. In Patients with Membranous Lupus Nephritis, Exostosin-Positivity and Exostosin-Negativity Represent Two Different Phenotypes. Journal of the American Society of Nephrology. 2021;:ASN.2020081181.

[14] Caza T, Hassen S, Dvanajscak Z, Kuperman M, Edmondson R, Herzog C, et al. NELL1 is a target antigen in malignancy-associated membranous nephropathy. Kidney Int [Internet]. 2020; Available from: https://doi.org/10.1016/j.kint.2020.07.039

[15] Picken MM. Proteomics and mass spectrometry in the diagnosis of renal amyloidosis. Clin Kidney J. 2015;8(6):665-672.

[16] Vogel C, Marcotte EM. Insights into the regulation of protein abundance from proteomic and transcriptomic analyses. Nat Rev Genet. 2012;13(4):227-232.

[17] Ralph DK, Matsen FA. Consistency of VDJ rearrangement and substitution parameters enables accurate B cell receptor sequence annotation. PLoS Comput Biol. 2016;12(1):1-25.

[18] Collins AM, Jackson KJL. A temporal model of human IgE and IgG antibody function. Front Immunol. 2013;4(AUG):1-6.

[19] Na W, Yi K, Song YS, Park MH. Dissecting the relationships of IgG subclasses and complements in membranous lupus nephritis and idiopathic membranous nephropathy. PLoS One. 2017;12(3):1-14.

[20] Bruhns P. Properties of mouse and human IgG receptors and their contribution to disease models. Blood. 2012;119(24):5640-5649.

[21] Murtas C, Bruschi M, Candiano G, Moroni G, Magistroni R, Magnano A, et al. Coexistence of different circulating anti-podocyte antibodies in membranous nephropathy. Clin J Am Soc Nephrol. 2012;7(9): 1394-1400.

[22] Ravindran A, Madden B, Charlesworth MC, Sharma R, Sethi A, Debiec H, et al. Proteomic analysis of complement proteins in membranous nephropathy. Kidney Int Reports [Internet]. 2020;5(5):618-626. Available from: https://doi.org/10.1016/j.ekir.2020.01.018

[23] Bomback AS, Markowitz GS, Appel GB. Complement-mediated glomerular diseases: A tale of 3 pathways. Kidney Int Reports [Internet]. 2016;1(3):148-155. Available from: http://dx.doi.org/10.1016/j.ekir.2016.06.005

[24] Jha V, Ganguli A, Saha TK, Kohli HS, Sud K, Gupta KL, et al. A randomized, controlled trial of steroids and cyclophosphamide in adults with nephrotic syndrome caused by idiopathic membranous nephropathy. J Am Soc Nephrol. 2007;18(6):1899-1904.

[25] Fernández-Juárez G, Rojas-Rivera J, Logt A-E van de, Justino J, Sevillano A, Caravaca-Fontán F, et al. The STARMEN trial indicates that alternating treatment with corticosteroids and cyclophosphamide is superior to sequential treatment with tacrolimus and rituximab in primary membranous nephropathy. Kidney Int [Internet]. 2020; Available from: https://doi.org/10.1016/j.kint.2020.10.014

[26] Fervenza FC, Appel GB, Barbour SJ, Rovin BH, Lafayette RA, Aslam N, et al. Rituximab or cyclosporine in the treatment of membranous nephropathy. N Engl J Med. 2019;381(1):36-46.

[27] Ponticelli C, Zucchelli P, Passerini P, Cesana B, Locatelli F, Pasquali S, et al. A 10-year follow-up of a randomized study with methylprednisolone and chlorambucil in membranous nephropathy. Kidney Int. 1995;48(5): 1600-1604.

[28] Appel G, Nachman P, Hogan S, Rodhakrishnan J, Old C,Herbert L, Fevrenza F, Kumor K, Petro B, Li L, Hardman J. Eculizumab (C5 complement inhibitor) in the treatment of idiopathic membranous nephropathy (abstract). J Am Soc Nephrol. 2002;13:668A-1857.

[29] Hayashi N, Okada K, Matsui Y, Fujimoto K, Adachi H, Yamaya H, et al. Glomerular mannose-binding lectin deposition in intrinsic antigen-related membranous nephropathy. Nephrol Dial Transplant. 2018;33(5):832-840.

[30] Bally S, Debiec H, Ponard D, Dijoud F, Rendu J, Fauré J, et al. Phospholipase A2 receptor-related

membranous nephropathy and mannan-binding lectin deficiency. J Am Soc Nephrol. 2016;27(12):3539-3544.

[31] Costa DMDN, Valente LM, Vajgel Fernandes G, Sandrin-Garcia P, Da Cruz HLA, Crovella S, et al. Mannose-binding Lectin2 gene polymorphism and IgG4 in membranous nephropathy. Nephron. 2018;139(2):181-188.

[32] Beck LH, Fervenza FC, Beck DM, Bonegio RGB, Malik FA, Erickson SB, et al. Rituximab-induced depletion of anti-PLA2R autoantibodies predicts response in membranous nephropathy. J Am Soc Nephrol. 2011;22(8): 1543-1550.

[33] Sekula P, Li Y, Stanescu HC, Wuttke M, Ekici AB, Bockenhauer D, et al. Genetic risk variants for membranous nephropathy: Extension of and association with other chronic kidney disease aetiologies. Nephrol Dial Transplant. 2017;32(2):325-332.

[34] Xie J, Liu L, Mladkova N, Li Y, Ren H, Wang W. The genetic architecture of membranous nephropathy and its potential to improve non-invasive diagnosis. 2020,11:1600

[35] Tomas NM, Beck LH, Meyer-Schwesinger C, Seitz-Polski B, Ma H, Zahner G, et al. Thrombo spondin Type-1 domain-containing 7A in idiopathic membranous nephropathy. N Engl J Med. 2014;371(24):2277-2287.

[36] Laurence H. Beck Jr.PLA2R and THSD7A: Disparate paths to the same disease? J Am Soc Nephrol. 2017;28:2579-2589.

[37] Saeed M, Beggs ML, Walker PD, Larsen CP. PLA2R-associated membranous glomerulopathy is modulated by common variants in PLA2R1 and HLA-DQA1 genes. Genes Immun [Internet]. 2014;15(8):556-561. Available from: http://dx.doi.org/10.1038/gene.2014.50

[38] Ramachandran R, Kumar V, Kumar A, Yadav AK, Nada R, Kumar H, et al. PLA2R antibodies, glomerular PLA2R deposits and variations in PLA2R1 and HLA-DQA1 genes in primary membranous nephropathy in south Asians. Nephrol Dial Transplant. 2016;31(9):1486-1493.

[39] Le WB, Shi JS, Zhang T, Liu L, Qin HZ, Liang S, et al. HLA-DRB1∗15:01 and HLA-DRB3∗02:02 in PLA2R-related membranous nephropathy. J Am Soc Nephrol. 2017;28(5):1642-1650.

[40] Thiri M, Honda K, Kashiwase K, Mabuchi A, Suzuki H, Watanabe K, et al. High-density association mapping and interaction analysis of PLA2R1 and HLA regions with idiopathic membranous nephropathy in Japanese. Sci Rep. 2016;6(November):1-8.

[41] Liu YH, Chen CH, Chen SY, Lin YJ, Liao WL, Tsai CH, et al. Association of phospholipase A2 receptor 1 polymorphisms with idiopathic membranous nephropathy in Chinese patients in Taiwan. J Biomed Sci [Internet]. 2010;17(1):81. Available from: http://www.jbiomedsci.com/content/17/1/81

[42] Bullich G, Ballarín J, Oliver A, Ayasreh N, Silva I, Santín S, et al. HLA-DQA1 and PLA2R1 polymorphisms and risk of idiopathic membranous nephropathy. Clin J Am Soc Nephrol. 2014;9(2):335-343.

[43] Nephropathy M. Related Articles : Copyright / Drug Dosage / Disclaimer. 2021;2021.

[44] Thibaudin D, Thibaudin L, Berthoux P, Mariat C, De Filippis JP, Laurent B, et al. TNFA2 and d2 alleles of the tumor necrosis factor alpha gene polymorphism are associated with

onset/occurrence of idiopathic membranous nephropathy. Kidney Int [Internet]. 2007;71(5):431-437. Available from: http://dx.doi.org/10.1038/sj.ki.5002054

[45] Use of pentoxifylline in membranous nephropathy in normal and malignant colon tissue. Lancet. 2001;357:1672-1673.

[46] Giacomelli M, Kumar R, Tampella G, Ceffa S, Bontempelli M. IL-4, IL-10 and TNF-<i>α</i> polymorphisms in idiopathic membranous nephropathy (IMN). Open J Immunol. 2015;05(05):233-243.

[47] KDGIO. Kdigo Clinical Practice Guideline on Glomerular Diseases. 2020;(June). Available from: https://kdigo.org/wp-content/uploads/2017/02/KDIGO-GN-GL-Public-Review-Draft_1-June- 2020.pdf.

[48] Chen CH, Chen SY, Shu KH, Wen MC, Cheng CH, Wu MJ, et al. Urokinase gene 3′-UTR T/C polymorphism is associated with malignancy and ESRD in idiopathic membranous nephropathy. Biomed Res Int. 2014;2014.

[49] Chen CH, Shu KH, Wen MC, Chen KJ, Cheng CH, Lian J Da, et al. Impact of plasminogen activator inhibitor-1 gene polymorphisms on primary membranous nephropathy. Nephrol Dial Transplant. 2008;23(10):3166-3173.

[50] Zhang H, Dong P, Yang X, Liu Z. Is Associated With Coronary Artery Disease Risk : a Meta-Analysis Commonly Studied Functional Variant in the. 2014;7(10):3777-3788.

[51] Conti F, Spinelli FR, Truglia S, Miranda F, Alessandri C, Ceccarelli F, et al. Kidney expression of toll like receptors in lupus nephritis: Quantification and Clinicopathological correlations. Mediators Inflamm. 2016;2016.

[52] Chen YT, Wei CC, Ng KL, Chen CH, Chan CJ, Chen XX, et al. Toll-like receptor 9 SNPs are susceptible to the development and progression of membranous glomerulonephritis: 27 years follow-up in Taiwan. Ren Fail. 2013;35(10):1370-1375.

[53] Chen SY, Chen WC, Chen YH, Chen CH, Huang YC, Huang PH, et al. Association of toll-like receptor 4 gene polymorphisms with primary membranous nephropathy in a high prevalence renal disease area in Taiwan. ScienceAsia. 2010;36(2):130-136.

[54] Kopp JB. Glomerular pathology in autosomal dominant MYH9 spectrum disorders: What are the clues telling us about disease mechanism. Kidney Int [Internet]. 2010;78(2):130-133. Available from: http://dx.doi.org/10.1038/ki.2010.82

[55] Chena YT, Chenc CH, Yend CH, Chena SY, Tsai FJ. Association between MYH9 gene polymorphisms and membranous glomerulonephritis patients in Taiwan. ScienceAsia. 2013;39(6):625-630.

[56] Westra H-J, Peters MJ, Esko T, Yaghootkar H, Schurmann C, Kettunen J, et al. Systematic identification of trans eQTLs as putative drivers of known disease associations. Nat Genet. 2013;45(10):1238-1243.

[57] Astle WJ, Elding H, Jiang T, Allen D, Ruklisa D, Mann AL, et al. The Allelic landscape of human blood cell trait variation and links to common complex disease. Cell. 2016;167(5):1415-1429.e19.

[58] Grumont RJ, Gerondakis S. Rel induces interferon regulatory factor 4 (IRF-4) expression in lymphocytes: modulation of interferon-regulated gene expression by rel/nuclear factor kappaB. J Exp Med. 2000;191(8):1281-1292.

Chapter 3

Influence Engulfment Cell Motility-1 (ELMO-1) Protein and Matrix Metalloproteases-9 (MMP-9) in Diabetic Nephropathy Patients

Elfiani Elfiani and Huntari Harahap

Abstract

Engulfment and Cell Motility-1 (ELMO-1) are well-known genes in Asia that can cause diabetic nephropathy in people with Diabetes Mellitus type-2. The increase in ELMO-1 protein affects Matrix Metalloproteases-9 (MMP-9) levels, both of which can cause chronic glomerular injury through dysregulation of Extra Cellular Matrix metabolism and decreased adhesive properties of endothelial cells to kidney structures. This study aims to prove differences in ELMO-1 and MMP-9 protein levels in type-2 Diabetes Mellitus (DM) patients with Diabetic Nephropathy compared to those without Diabetic Nephropathy. This study is a comparative observational study with venous blood samples taken from 60 patients with type-2 DM patients without Diabetic Nephropathy as a control and type-2 DM group with Diabetic Nephropathy cases diagnosed based on the criteria of Glomerular Filtration Rate and Albumin-to-Creatinine Ratio. In this study, the levels of ELMO-1 and MMP-9 proteins were checked by ELISA (Enzyme-linked Immunosorbent Assay). The results showed that the mean plasma ELMO-1 value was higher in the Diabetes Mellitus type-2 group with Diabetic Nephropathy than without the Diabetic Nephropathy group (t-test, $p = 0.025$). The mean plasma MMP-9 value was higher in the DM with Diabetic Nephropathy group rather than in the DM without Diabetic Nephropathy group (t-test, $p = 0.032$). Conclusion ELMO-1 and MMP-9 levels were higher in Diabetes Mellitus type-2 with diabetic nephropathy.

Keywords: Diabetic Nephropathy, Diabetes Mellitus, Engulfment and Cell Motility-1, Matrix Metalloproteases-9, chronic glomerular injury, dysregulation of ECM metabolism, Albumin to Creatinine Ratio, Glomerular Filtration Rate

1. Introduction

The prevalence of Diabetes Mellitus (DM) increases globally; in 2011, about 366 million people experienced Diabetes, and it is estimated to continue to grow to 522 million people in 2030 [1]. Diabetes Mellitus will cause damage and failure of various organs; one of these organs is the kidney. This complication of DM in the kidney is called Diabetic Nephropathy. The prevalence of Diabetic Nephropathy occurs in 20–40% of all type-2 DM patients [2]. Kidney damage in Diabetic Nephropathy is irreversible and causes an increase in morbidity, mortality, and the burden of health financing in most countries [3].

The principal risks of Diabetic Nephropathy are modifiable, namely blood pressure, blood sugar, and dyslipidemia. Meanwhile, factors that cannot be modified include age, race, and genetic profile [4]. However, the pathogenesis that contributes to Diabetic Nephropathy incidence is not fully understood, especially the role of genetics [5]. So that efforts to obtain genetic information in type-2 DM patients who are susceptible/at risk of Diabetic Nephropathy provide an opportunity to predict and diagnose this complication early [6].

The ELMO-1 gene is a functional gene that codes for the formation of the ELMO-1 protein, located on chromosome 7 of mammalian cells. ELMO-1 protein helps engulf "eating" or clean apoptotic cells and plays a role in cell motility and cell shape changes [7, 8].

ELMO-1 protein increases in hyperglycemic conditions and TGF-β1 (Tumor Growth Factor Beta-1), collagen type-1, fibronectin expression, and Extra Cellular Matrix (ECM) in the kidneys. MMP-9 also plays a vital role in diabetic nephropathy. Increased secretion of MMP-9 destroys the podocyte diaphragm, which is an essential component in maintaining the standard barrier of glomerular filtration [10].

2. Diabetic nephropathy

2.1 Research methods and study design

This study is an observational study with a cross-sectional comparative study design. This study was conducted at three hospitals in Jambi Province, Indonesia, with a total sample of 60 people. Control this research is Diabetes Mellitus type 2 group without Diabetic Nephropathy patients diagnosed with type-2 Diabetes without impaired kidney function and two times the value examination, Albumin to Creatinine Ratio (ACR) <30 mg/g for 2–3 months mild/normal albuminuria levels. Diabetes mellitus with nephropathy diabetes has hemodialysis, decreased Glomerular Filtration Rate, and or persistent albuminuria.

The inclusion criteria in this study were over 20 years ago, had suffered from type-2 Diabetes for at least five years, had a medical record with routine laboratory examination data in the form of blood sugar and urinalysis, assessment of kidney function (urea levels and creatinine), ultrasound, and ACR examination at least two times in 3–6 months and were willing to participate in this study by signing the informed consent. Exclusion criteria in this study were patients with urinary tract infections, other kidney diseases such as kidney stones and kidney cysts (from medical records), pregnancy, and patients with autoimmune or immunocompromised diseases.

ELMO-1 and MMP-9 levels were examined using ELISA (Enzyme-linked Immunosorbent Assay). Sample this research from blood plasma; then carried out according to the ELISA kit instructions for human ELMO-1 from MyBioSource catalog number MBS9321199 and MMP-9 from RayBioR catalog number ELH-MMP9.

This research has passed ethics from the Faculty of Medicine's research ethics commission team, Andalas University, and received ethical clearance number 706/KEP/FK/2019. Data analysis used a t-test because the data distribution was normal.

2.2 Results

2.2.1 Basic characteristics of research subjects

The basic characteristics of the assessed research subjects are shown in **Table 1**.

Based on the essential characteristics of research subjects, it is known that Type-2 Diabetes with Diabetic Nephropathy has systolic and diastolic blood pressure, fasting blood sugar levels, and blood sugar levels 2 hours after eating. Albumin to creatinine ratio (ACR) in urine is higher than non-diabetic nephropathy. And statistically significant. In contrast, the mean value of glomerular filtration rate (GFR) was lower in the Diabetic Nephropathy group and statistically significant.

2.2.2 Levels of plasma protein ELMO-1 and MMP-9

ELMO-1 and MMP-9 protein levels between DM subjects with Diabetic Nephropathy and without Diabetic Nephropathy are presented in **Tables 2** and **3** below.

Table 2 shows that the mean ELMO-1 plasma value was higher in the DM group with Diabetic Nephropathy and without Diabetic Nephropathy group, statistically significant ($p < 0.05$).

Table 3 shows that the mean plasma MMP-9 value was higher in the DM group with Diabetic Nephropathy than the without Diabetic Nephropathy group. And this difference was statistically significant ($p = 0.032$).

2.3 Discussion

The Genome-Wide Association Studies in Japan in 2005 identified the part of Engulfment and cell motility-1 (ELMO-1) in diabetic nephropathy. A study using

Characteristics	Diabetes with Diabetic Nephropathy (n = 30)	Diabetes without Diabetic Nephropathy (n = 30)	p-value
Age	51,17 ± 7,88	49,87 ± 8,42	0,539[a]
Gender			
Male, n Female, n	15 (57,7%) 15 (44,1%)	11 (36,7%) 19 (55,9%)	0,297[b]
Fasting blood sugar levels	160,40 ± 60,32	138,90 ± 35,54	0,249[a]
Blood sugar levels 2 hours after eating	245,87 ± 59,57	237,27 ± 84,56	0,428[a]
Systolic blood pressure	139,33 ± 17,21	122,43 ± 14,47	**<0,001**[a,*]
Diastolic blood pressure	83,33 ± 9,59	78,00 ± 8,87	**<0,033**[a,*]
Urine creatinine	95,64 ± 72,65	89,59 ± 71,53	0,887[a]
Urine albumin	618,83 ± 876,23	12,67 ± 9,65	**<0,001**[a,*]
Albumin to creatinine ratio	1387,67 ± 2743,37	14,21 ± 6,6	**<0,001**[a,*]
Glomerular filtration rate, mL/min	69,76 ± 36,10	92,91 ± 23,76	**0,005**[a]

[a]*t-test.*
[b]*Chi-square test.*
[*]*Statistically significant; p-value < 0,05.*

Table 1.
Basic characteristics of research subjects.

Protein	Diabetes with Diabetic Nephropathy (n = 30)	Diabetes without Diabetic Nephropathy (n = 30)	p-value
Plasma ELMO-1 (ng/mL)	623,83 ± 940,73	211,21 ± 209,98	**0,025**[a,*]

[a]*t-test.*
[*]*p-value <0,05; statistically significant (p < 0,05).*

Table 2.
ELMO-1 plasma levels between DM subjects with diabetic nephropathy and without diabetic nephropathy.

Protein	Diabetes with ND (n = 30)	Diabetes with ND non-ND (n = 30)	p-value
Plasma MMP-9 (pg/mL)	1800,14 ± 1871,18	981,79 ± 758,49	**0,032**[a,*]

[a]*t-test.*
**p-value <0,05; statistically significant.*

Table 3.
Plasma levels of MMP-9 between DM subjects with ND and non-ND.

diabetic rats found that increased ELMO-1 protein levels were in diabetic kidneys compared to normal rats [9]. Functions ELMO-1 proteins were phagocytosis of apoptotic cells and cell motility in mammals [7]. Failure to clear apoptotic cells can cause inflammation and autoimmunity damage [8].

In this study, there was no difference in age and gender. Because due to the nine samples' consecutive sampling technique, where there is a balanced age range between the case and control groups. There is a difference in age characteristics in the literature, stating that diabetic nephropathy is more common in old age. Because it is associated with a longer duration of disease in old age, and diabetes mellitus has been more than five years [11].

Based on patient characteristics, it is known that the mean value of glomerular filtration rate is lower in the diabetic group with Diabetic Nephropathy compared without Diabetic Nephropathy. This situation is because, in diabetic nephropathy, there is a more severe decrease in kidney function. The reduction in glomerular hydration rate in type-II DM patients is proportional to the degree of albuminuria. The more significant the reduction in glomerular filtration rate, the heavier the degree of albuminuria [11, 12].

In this study, the Diabetic Nephropathy group had a higher average blood pressure than non-ND Diabetes Mellitus. Blood pressure decreases the rate of glomerular psychopathy and albuminuria in Diabetic Nephropathy [13, 14]. The elevated blood pressure in diabetic nephropathy occurred due to disruption of the Renin-Angiotensin-Aldosterone System (RAA's) and decreased renal blood flow [13, 14].

In the study, ELMO-1 protein levels were higher in patients with diabetic nephropathy. ELMO-1 protein contributed to chronic glomerular injury progression through the increased accumulation of the extracellular matrix and decreased cell adhesion [14]. The extracellular matrix accumulation causes thickening of the glomerulus and renal tubules, a marker of advanced diabetes nephropathy [13].

This study reported higher plasma ELMO-1 and MMP-9 levels in diabetic patients with ND and was statistically significant (**Tables 2** and **3**). Functional studies on cultured cells and experimental animals show the role of the ELMO-1 protein in ND. Previous research has shown an increase in ELMO-1 signal with the in situ hybridization (FISH) method in the kidney of rats with nephropathy compared to those without nephropathy.

MMP-9 protein is a protein involved in the degradation of the extracellular matrix and glomerular turnover. Changes in MMP-9 expression are associated with the development of diabetic nephropathy. Hyperglycemia, an increase in advanced glycation end products, and oxidative stress that occurs in people with Diabetes increase the expression of MMP-9. MMP-9 protein cause of disrupts the integrity and increases the permeability of podocytes to albumin, and increases protein synthesis, which is involved in forming the extracellular matrix. All of these are processes that occur in Diabetes nephropathy [10, 15, 16].

3. Conclusion

Engulfment and Cell Motility-1 (ELMO-1) and Matrix Metalloproteases-9 (MMP-9) protein levels were higher in Diabetic Nephropathy compared to Diabetes Mellitus without Diabetic Nephropathy and difference was statistically significant. Required a larger number of samples and performed prospectively.

Acknowledgements

Thanks to the Faculty of Medicine and Health Sciences, Jambi University and the Raden Mattaher Jambi Regional General Hospital, the Baiturrahim Jambi Pertamedika Hospital, the Jambi MMC (Mayang Medical Center) Hospital for research.

Appendix and nomenclature

ACR	Albumin-to-Creatinine Ratio
ACEI	Angiotensin Enzyme Inhibitor
ADA	American Diabetes Association
DM	Diabetes Mellitus
ECM	Extra Cellular Matrix
ELISA	Enzyme-linked Immunosorbent Assay
ELMO-1	Engulfment and cell motility-1
IDF	International Diabetes Federation
MMP	Matrix Metalloproteases

Author details

Elfiani Elfiani[1*] and Huntari Harahap[2]

1 Department of Internal Medicine, Raden Mattaher Hospital Jambi, Jambi, Indonesia

2 Department of Physiology, Faculty of Medicine and Health Sciences, Jambi University, Jambi, Indonesia

*Address all correspondence to: elfiani@gmail.com

References

[1] Whiting DR., Guariguata L., Weil C., Shaw J., 2011. IDF Diabetes Atlas: Global Estimates of the Prevalence of Diabetes for 2011 and 2030. Diabetes Reseach Clinical Practice 94: 311 – 321.

[2] Kim SS., Kim JH., Kim IJ., 2016. Current Challenges in Diabetic Nephropathy: Early Diagnostic and Way to Improve Outcomes. Endocrinol Metab 31; 245-253

[3] Lim AK., 2014. Diabetic nephropathy–Complications and treatment. International Journal of Nephrology and Renovascular Disease 7: 361-381

[4] Gogolin, K. et al., 2005. Assessment of 115 Candidate Genes for Diabetic Nephropathy by Transmission/ Disequilibrium Test. NCBI.

[5] Conserva F., Gesualdo L., Papale M., 2015. A Systems Biology Overview on Human Diabetic Nephropathy: From Genetic Susceptibility to Post-Transcriptional and Post-Translational Modifications. Journal of Diabetes Research Article ID7934504 23pages http://dx.doi.org/10.1155/2016/7934504

[6] Lin CH., Chang YC., Chuang LM., 2016. Early detection of diabetic kidney disease: Present limitations and future perspectives. World J Diabetes 7(14): 290-301

[7] Gumienny TL., Brugnera E., Tosello-Trampont AC., Kinchen JM., Haney LB., Nishiwaki K., Walk SF., Nemergut ME., Macara IG., Francis R., 2001. CED-12/ELMO, a novel member of the CrkI I/Dock180/Rac pathway, is required for phagocytosis and cell migration. Cell. 107:27-41.

[8] Ravichandran SK., 2007. Engulfment of apoptotic cells: signals for a good meal. NCBI.

[9] Shimazaki A., Kawamura Y., Kanazawa A., Sekine A., Saito S., Tsunoda T., Koya D., Babazono T., Tanaka Y., Matsuda M., Kawai K., Iiizumi T., Imanishi M., Shinosaki T., Yanagimoto T., Ikeda M., Omachi S., Kashiwagi A., Kaku K., Iwamoto Y., Kawamori R., Kikkawa R., Nakajima M., Nakamaru Y., Maeda S., 2005. Genetic Variations in the Gen Encoding ELMO1 Are Associated With Susceptibility to Diabetic Nephropathy. Diabetes 54: 1171-1178.

[10] Li SY., Po-Huang H., Yang AH., Tarng DC., Yang WC., Lin CC., Chen JW., Scho¨nbein GS., Lin SJ., 2014. Matrix metalloproteinase-9 deficiency attenuates diabetic nephropathy by modulation of podocyte functions and dedifferentiation. Kidney International. 86: 358-369.

[11] Gheith O, Farouk N, Nampoory N, Halim MA, Al-otaibi T, 2016. Diabetic kidney disease: world wide difference of prevalence and risk factor. J Nephropharmacol 5(1): 49-56.

[12] Retnakaran R., Cull CA., Thorne KI., Adler AI., Holman RR., 2006. Risk Factors for Renal Dysfunction in Type 2 Diabetes UK Prospective Diabetes study 74. Diabetes 55: 1832-1839.

[13] Alicic RZ, Rooney MT, Tuttle KR, 2017. Diabetic Kidney Disease Challenges, Progress and Possibilities. Clin J Am Soc Nephrol 12: 2023-2045.

[14] Shimazaki A., Tanaka Y., Shinosaki T., 2006. ELMO1 increases expression of extracellular matrix proteins and inhibits cell adhesion to ECMs. Kidney International *70,* 1769-1776.

[15] Xu X., Xiao L., Xiao P., Yang S., Chen G., Liu F., Kanwar YY., Sun L.,

2014. A Glimpse of Matrix Metalloproteinase in Diabetic Nephropathy. Curr Med Chem 21(28): 3244-3260.

[16] Thrailkill KM., Bunn RC., Fowlkes JL., 2009. Matrix metallo proteinases: their potential role in the pathogenesis of diabetic nephropathy. *Endocrine* 35(1): 1-10.

Chapter 4

Therapeutic Apheresis in Renal Transplantation: Indications and Strategies

Jean Jeanov Filipov and Emil Paskalev Dimitrov

Abstract

Kidney transplantation (KT) is the best renal replacement therapy in patients with chronic kidney disease (CKD). However, its success is limited due to insufficient number of donors worldwide and graft or patient loss. A major cause for poorer graft survival is donor-specific antibodies (DSAs). Therapeutic apheresis (TA) is a well-recognized option for increasing the donor pool by treating HLA-sensitized patients and making AB0-incompatible KT possible. In addition, its use in patients with DSA has beneficial effect on graft survival. The aim of our review is to demonstrate the current knowledge on the use of TA (plasma exchange and immunoadsorption) in KT. In addition to the current guidelines, new trends in TA use prior to and after KT will be reviewed.

Keywords: therapeutic apheresis, kidney transplantation, desensitization, AB0 incompatible transplantation, plasma exchange, immunoadsorption

1. Introduction

Kidney transplantation is a type of renal replacement therapy (RRT) in patients with end-stage renal disease (ESRD), which is associated with the best patient outcomes. A major breakthrough was detected with the introduction of cyclosporine A in the immunosuppressive regimen. One-year survival improved further more with the use of novel immunosuppression (tacrolimus and mycophenolate), with graft survival rates for the first year after KT surpassing 95%. Despite the amazing results over the years, several problems are still unsolved.

A major obstacle to the success of KT is the shortage of donors worldwide [1]. An additional cause for donor insufficiency is the presence of donor-specific HLA antibodies (DSAs) in ESRD patients. HLA sensitization is caused mainly by blood transfusions, pregnancy, and previous organ transplantation. DSAs are associated with increased risk for acute rejection and poorer graft survival [2].

Another option to increase donor options could be AB0-incompatible transplantation. However, in these cases the innate blood group barrier should be overcome in order to avoid hyperacute rejection.

Finally, long-term graft survival (at the fifth and tenth year after KT) is significantly lower, compared to short-term one. One of explanations for this finding is the development of de novo DSA, which in turn are related to antibody-mediated rejection and poorer graft survival [3].

IntechOpen

Therapeutic apheresis (TA) is a method by which pathological elements of the immune system (cells, antibodies, and immune complexes) are being removed via extracorporeal system, thus influencing disease activity. Different TA techniques have been developed over the years. The most important ones in organ transplantation are plasma exchange (PEX) and immunoadsorption (IA).

1.1 Types of TA in kidney transplantation

1.1.1 Plasma exchange (PEX)

PEX is an invasive therapeutic method, separating plasma from blood cells. Thus pathogenic antibodies or other large molecules are removed and plasma is replaced by human albumin and/or fresh frozen plasma (FFP). The blood is pumped out of patient's circulation, and is transferred to a separator (centrifugal bowl or hollow fiber membrane), separating plasma from blood cells. Afterward blood cells are pumped into patient's vein and patient's plasma is substituted by protein solution (human albumin and/or FFP). Generally, central venous catheter is used as vascular access, though arteriovenous fistulas and large peripheral veins can also be used. The mechanism of action of PEX is removal of pathogenic antibodies, substitution of plasma proteins, and modification of cell response. However, the procedure is associated with albumin and fibrinogen loss, the latter being linked to increased bleeding risk. Therefore, more selective techniques for antibody removal were developed. A subset of PEX is the selective PEX, in which a special membrane plasma separator with smaller pores is used. Its use in renal transplantation currently is limited.

1.1.2 Double filtration plasmapheresis (DFPP)

DFPP is a semi-selective separation technique, based on membrane PEX. After initial separation of plasma from blood cells, additional filtration of plasma is performed with different diameter of fiber pores, so that target protein fractions are filtered and the rest are returned into the circulation. This technique showed up to 70% reduction in albumin loss after the procedure lower risk for infections and allergic reactions. The method was used initially for ABo-incompatible transplantation [4].

1.1.3 Cryofiltration

The technique was designed to remove cryoglobulins in several immune diseases. After plasma is initially filtrated, it is cooled to 4°C. This causes precipitation of cryoglobulins and they do not pass the second membrane. Afterward, the cooled plasma is warmed to body temperature again and is returned to the patient. The method was used in AB0-incompatible transplantation and HLA-sensitized patients. However, further studies are needed to incorporate cryofiltration in transplantation practice [5, 6].

1.1.4 Selective adsorption, immunoadsorption

In selective adsorption the plasma is filtered at the first step of the procedure, and at the second stage the initial filtrate runs through pre-arranged immunosorbents. Thus specific antibodies can be selectively removed, whereas albumin and clotting factors are returned to the patient. There are two types of selective adsorption—*immunoadsorbtion (IA)* and *selective plasma adsorption*. In IA either the plasma runs through column bearing antigens directed against certain antibody, or antibodies against certain plasma constituents. In selective plasma adsorption plasma components are removed by binding to ligands other than antibodies and antigens (e.g., heparin and dextransulfate in LDL adsorption).

Practically only IA is used in transplantology. There are different IA techniques according to IA devices [7]:

1. IA using immobilized antibodies—sheep polyclonal anti-human IgG antibodies are used to remove IgG antibodies from plasma

2. IA using immobilized antigens and synthetic epitopes—the IA columns contain only immobilized antigens/epitopes, thus removing the pathogenic antibodies only. This method is the most specific one.

3. IA using staphylococcal protein A—IA columns containing immobilized Staphylococcal protein A, which effectively clears IgG types 1,2, and 4 by binding their Fc portions

1.1.5 Extracorporeal photopheresis (ECP)

ECP is a method, in which white blood cells are separated from plasma and are being treated extracorporeally with 8-methoxypsoralen (8-MOP) followed by exposure to ultraviolet A (UVA) light. The treated cells are then returned into patient's circulation. Initially used in the treatment of T-cell lymphoma, its indications have expanded in solid organ transplantation (heart, lung, and kidney). In renal transplantation ECP was used in recurrent and refractory rejection, as well as in antibody-mediated chronic rejection with conflicting results [7].

1.2 TA immunosuppression in KT

PEX and IA can remove the already produced antibodies, but they cannot influence the antibody production. However, after TA a rise in antibody formation and increase in B-cell proliferation occurs [8]. Therefore, TA should be coupled with adequate immunosuppression. In TA prior to or after renal transplantation the most widely used immunosuppressive medications are the biological agents—Thymoglobulin (ATG, dose 1–1.5 mg/kg, different protocols exist), Rituximab (standard dose 375 mg/m^2/weekly for 2–4 weeks) and intravenous immunoglobulins (IVIG, 100 mg/kg after each procedure). Eculizumab is also taken into consideration in high-risk patients prior to and after KT. Its effectivity is fully recognized in post-transplant atypical hemolytic uremic syndrome (aHUS). Further trials are needed to evaluate the exact place of this monoclonal drug in transplantation [9]. In addition, as the KT in sensitized patients is regarded as high-risk procedure, anti-CD25 agents can also be applied.

1.3 Classification of TA according to effectivity

The beneficial effect of TA is difficult to assess due to the relatively low number of randomized controlled trials (RCTs). According to the American Society for Apheresis (ASFA) the indications for TA have been classified into four categories, according to the possible beneficial effect of the procedure [10]:

- Category 1—Disorders for which apheresis is accepted as first-line therapy, either as a primary standalone treatment or in conjunction with other modes of treatment, for example, recurrent focal segmental glomerulosclerosis (FSGS).

- Category 2—Disorders for which apheresis is accepted as second-line therapy, either as a standalone treatment or in conjunction with other modes of treatment, for example, antibody-mediated rejection (AMR) in AB0-incompatible KT.
- Category 3—Optimum role of apheresis therapy is not established. Decision-making should be individualized—for example, HLA desensitization in deceased donation in AB0-compatible transplantation.
- Category 4—Disorders in which published evidence demonstrates or suggests apheresis to be ineffective or harmful—for example, lupus nephritis.

2. TA prior to renal transplantation

The presence of antibodies against donor HLA alleles significantly increases the risk for acute rejection and graft survival. Similarly, AB0-incompatible KT is associated with hyperacute rejection due to the presence of antibodies against A-/B-antigens on the surface of vascular endothelial cells. Therapeutic apheresis plays a key role in reducing the titers of pathogenic antibodies, thus significantly improving graft survival, reduces the risk for graft rejection, and increases the chances for successful KT.

2.1 AB0-incompatible (AB0i) KT

The antigens, associated with AB0 blood groups are expressed not only on the red blood cell's membrane, but also on the surface of the endothelial cells, making the A-/B-glycolipids one of the most important antigens, related to transplantation immunology. The naturally circulating antibodies against the above-mentioned AB0 antigens in AB0i renal transplantation lead to hyperacute rejection, severe endothelial damage, and thrombosis, which finally leads to graft loss within minutes after revascularization. Therefore, AB0 incompatibility is a major obstacle to successful KT. It was estimated, that its treatment can effectively increase the numbers of living donors by up to 30%. In addition, the current protocols for AB0i KT demonstrate comparable success to AB0-compatible KT [11].

Different protocols for desensitization in AB0i KT exist, generally most of them aim for target post-procedure isoagglutinin titers ≤1:8 (**Table 1**, [12–14]). In the early stages of AB0i KT splenectomy was performed in addition to PA. However, this practice was abandoned due to the risk for infectious complications and immunosuppressive agents were introduced in everyday practice. In cases, in which PEX was used, substitution with albumin or FFP is needed. FFP should be both donor and recipient AB0 compatible [10]. The number of procedures varies according to baseline isoagglutinin titers. The most widely used TA techniques are PEX and selective IA, though DFPP can also be taken into consideration (**Table 1**). As TA markedly improves prognosis in AB0i KT, it is regarded as first-line therapy in AB0i recipient-donor pairs (ASFA category 1) [10].

2.2 HLA desensitization

The presence of antibodies against the HLA alleles of the donor prior to KT is another obstacle for the success of the procedure. The presence of donor-specific anti-HLA antibodies (DSAs) cause graft loss due to antibody-mediated rejection (AbMR) and is also referred as HLA-incompatible (HLAi) KT. At higher titers DSA

Target antibody level at KT day	TA strategy	Immunosuppression	Results	Reference
1:8 initial phase, later 1:32	PEX 30 ml/kg/ session, alternate days, start 7 days prior to KT	RTX 200 mg on day (−15); IVIG 5 g after each PEX (total 10–25 g), Thymoglobulin—two doses, total 3 mg/kg	1 year graft and patient survival 97.8%	Ray DS et al.
1:8	DFPP start: 7 days prior to KT, alternate days, performed post KT	RTX at day −14 Tac and mycophenolate at day (-7)	Graft survival 87%, patient survival 93%, post-transplant infection rate 13%	Jha PK et al
1:8	Antigen-specific IA Start: day (-6) four sessions, treatment volume: two plasma volumes After KT three more sessions within nine days	RTX 375 mg/m^2—day (-14) Triple immunosuppression (Tac, MMF, Prednisolone) IVIG 0.5 g/kg after final IA	All patients had good graft function during the follow-up	Tydén G et al

TA—therapeutic apheresis, PEX—plasma exchange, DFFP—double filtration plasmapheresis, IA—immunoadsorption, RTX—rituximab, IVIG—intravenous immunoglobulin, Tac—tacrolimus, MMF—mycophenolate mofetil.

Table 1.
Desensitization protocols in ABo incompatible kidney transplantation.

cause hyperacute AbMR, whereas lower titers result in acute or chronic AbMR [7]. The major causes for HLA sensitization are previous transplantation, blood transfusion, or pregnancy.

Due to the increased immunological risk, sensitized candidates remain significantly longer on the waiting list. It was estimated, that approximately 30% of the candidates for KT have detectable anti-HLA antibodies and half of them are highly sensitized, being sensitized to more than 80% of the possible HLA alleles. Desensitization protocols, by which undetectable DSA titers and negative cross-match are achieved, significantly improve graft survival, especially in living donation.

2.2.1 HLA desensitization in ABO-compatible KT, deceased donors

In deceased donor KT (DDKT) there are conflicting data considering the effectivity of TA. In patients on the waiting list, attempts have been made to perform HLA desensitization, with unclear benefit (**Table 2**, [15–21]). However, the prolonged exposure to immunosuppressive agents should be taken into consideration.

More studies have been performed in TA and DDKT in the perioperative setting. Generally, the aim is negative cross-match to be achieved prior to KT. Different protocols were suggested, using PEX/IA, accompanied by immunosuppressive agents (rituximab, IVIG, ATG). Though short-term results were encouraging, long-term ones are still conflicting [21]. AbMR and T-cell rejection had higher incidence in DSA/+/ kidney transplant recipients (KTRs), especially in those with higher mean intensity fluorescence (MFI) [19, 21]. Therefore, higher pre-transplant DSA titers have poorer prognosis, despite current desensitization protocols in deceased donors. Currently, due to the insufficient data on the use of TA in HLA desensitization in DDKT and the conflicting results it falls into category 3 of the latest ASFA guidelines [10].

TA on the waiting list				
Study design	**TA strategy**	**Immunosuppression**	**Results**	**Reference**
IA and immunosuppression in HLA-sensitized ESRD patients	IA	Cyclophosphamide + steroids	Unclear benefit, safe procedure	Hiesse C. et al
PEX and immunosuppression in HLA-sensitized ESRD patients	PEX—12 procedures	Cyclophosphamide + steroids on the first day of PP, tapered till KT	9 out of 23 lost grafts in the first 2 months post KT, 59% graft survival at fifth year post-transplant	Alarabi A. et al.
Peritransplant TA				
PEX in DDKT, positive cross-match, aiming negative one	PEX—1 procedure	RTX	First year graft survival 92.4%, patient survival 95.8%	Morath C et al.
Desensitization IVIG vs. IVIG/RTX/PEX, negative cross-match on KT day *Short-term results*	PEX—9 procedures, alternate days post KT	IVIG 2 g/kg on days 0,2,42, 63; RTX days 2 and 22	Better GFR and greater DSA-MFI decrease in IVIG/RTX/PEX group	Loupy et al.
Desensitization with IVIG/RTX/PEX MFI˃3000 vs. MFI 500–3000, both groups with negative cross-match on KT day *Long-term results*	PEX—9 procedures, alternate days post KT	IVIG 2 g/kg on days; 0,2,42, 63 RTX days 2 and 22	Similar GFR in both groups; lower incidence of T-cell rejection in MFI 500–3000	Amrouche L et al.
Desensitization in DDKT broadly sensitized patients; KT performed after negative cross-match achieved	IA (staphylococcal protein A) initial volume 6 L, later 2–3 plasma volumes; first session—immediately before KT; after KT—IA every 1–3 days, up to 7 weeks	ATG	Similar graft and patient survival compared to DSA/−/ at third year post KT	Bartel G. et al. The Vienna group
Extended previous study of the Vienna group, no change in protocol			Poorer graft survival compared to DSA/−/ at third year post KT, higher incidence of AbMR in DSA/+/, higher MFI was associated with higher risk for rejection	Schwaiger E et al. The Vienna group

TA—therapeutic apheresis, PEX—plasma exchange, IA—immunoadsorption, RTX—rituximab, IVIG—intravenous immunoglobulin, KT—kidney transplantation, DDKT—deceased donor kidney transplantation, MFI—mean intensity fluorescence, ATG—thymoglobulin, DSA—donor-specific antibodies, AbMR—antibody-mediated rejection, GFR—glomerular filtration rate, ESRD—end-stage renal disease.

Table 2.
HLA desensitization protocols in ABo-compatible deceased donors kidney transplantation.

2.2.2 HLA desensitization in ABO-compatible KT, living donors

HLA desensitization is far more important and more effective in living donor kidney transplantation (LDKT). A multicenter study demonstrated that KTRs with HLAi LDKT have better survival than patients on the waiting list without being transplanted or those on the waiting list with deceased donor KT. The benefit was significant in the short and in the long run [22].

The most used TA techniques in LDKT desensitization protocols are PEX and IA. Usually 4–8 sessions of PEX are performed prior to KT on alternate days. In most of the studies low-dose IVIG (10–150 mg/kg) was infused after each PEX, though the IVIG can be applied at the end of the series too [10]. Post-transplant PEX procedures were also performed (5–9 sessions) [22, 23]. In some studies mycophenolate and tacrolimus were added to the protocol 14 days prior to KT [23]. RTX was also used in certain protocols, forming a triple regimen—PEX/low-dose IVIG/RTX. Though an overall AbMR rate between 30 and 40% was detected, graft and patient survival reached up to 93 and 95% respectively at the first year [10, 24].

IA is the other most widely used TA modality in LDKT desensitization. It is coupled with RTX ± IVIG and graft survival rates reach up to 100% at the second year. Pre-transplant oral immunosuppressive agents could be used (tacrolimus + mycophenolate + steroids) and ATG/Basiliximab induction therapy as well [25].

2.3 Desensitization in combined HLAi/ABOi KT

In the rare setting of both HLAi and ABOi KT desensitization using PEX/IA plays a key role. A study using TA (PEX or specific/non-specific IA), combined with IVIG, two doses of RTX (375 mg/m^2) and Tacrolimus (0.2 mg/kg started 10 days prior to KT) demonstrated excellent graft and patient survival [26].

3. TA after renal transplantation

The major indications for TA after successful KT are AbMR and recurrent or de novo glomerular disease.

3.1 TA in AbMR

3.1.1 Acute AbMR

In HLA-desensitized patients AbMR ranges between 30 and 40% post-transplant, despite successful desensitization prior to KT. However, acute AbMR can occur in up to 10% after KT due to de novo DSA. The diagnosis is based on the presence of DSA, C4d deposition in peritubular capillaries, and evidence of tissue injury (typically associated with neutrophil/macrophage infiltration) [27]. However, AbMR without C4d deposition is also possible according to the BANFF criteria [28]. Acute AbMR is categorized into early (within 6 months after KT) and late (more 6 months after KT). Both types are associated with poorer graft survival; however, early acute AbMR is more responsive to the current treatment protocols.

PEX and IA play a key role in acute AbMR treatment and fall into ASFA category 1 [10]. The protocol consists usually of at least five TA procedures, coupled with IVIG infusion (total does 1–2 g/kg, 100–200 mg/kg after each procedure). In addition, RTX was tested as immunosuppressive agent, added to TA + IVIG combination. The results for RTX-based protocols so far are inconsistent, as some studies indicate benefit from the triple combination, whereas others fail to establish positive effect on short-term or long-term graft survival [29, 30].

Other preparations were tested in combination to TA as well: Bortezomib, complement component 1 (C1)—inhibitor and eculizumab (C5a inhibitor) currently with unclear benefit, indicating the need for further research in this field [31].

3.1.2 Hyperacute AbMR

Hyperacute AbMR presents with cyanosis and anuria, occurring minutes after revascularization of the graft, and is caused by pre-formed antibodies against the graft (AB0 incompatibility, HLA-DSA, antibodies against endothelial and monocyte antigens). It is currently a rare finding due to improved pre-transplant immunological evaluation. Histologically small vessel endothelial damage is detected, as well as thrombosis and neutrophil infiltration. There is no treatment, the only option is nephrectomy [32].

3.1.3 Chronic AbMR

Chronic AbMR is diagnosed by the presence of donor-specific antibodies, C4d deposition in peritubular capillaries, and evidence of chronic tissue injury. Chronic tissue injury encompasses duplication of the glomerular basement membrane (GBM), multilamination of the peritubular capillary basement membrane, arterial intimal fibrosis without elastosis, and interstitial fibrosis with tubular atrophy [27]. Though different TA techniques have been tested in chronic AbMR, including ECP, the procedure is generally ineffective due to the chronic histology findings [27].

3.1.4 De novo DSA and subclinical AbMR

The detection of de novo DSA after KT is associated with poorer transplant outcomes due to higher incidence of chronic allograft nephropathy (CAN) [33]. Subclinical AbMR is main cause for CAN in these cases. It presents with the typical histology and serology for AbMR, without significant changes in the laboratory and clinical findings. A recent study failed to demonstrate significant beneficial effect from two sessions of DFPP+RTX in subclinical AbMR. In this paper, patients with de novo DSA without data for rejection, who received no treatment, were also evaluated. In the follow-up period no significant changes in graft function and proteinuria in this subgroup occurred [34]. Therefore more clinical trials are needed to evaluate the importance of TA in subclinical AbMR and in de novo DSA without rejection.

3.1.5 TA in non-DSA post KT

The importance of non-DSA post KT is currently unclear. Though certain studies demonstrate association between non-DSA and acute AbMR, others fail to establish such relationship, even at MFI up to 10,000 [35, 36]. Additional trials are needed to fully evaluate the significance of non-DSA and the possible treatment methods in the future.

3.2 TA in recurrent disease

3.2.1 Recurrent focal segmental glomerulosclerosis (FSGS)

FSGS is a disease, in the pathogenesis of which an unidentified plasma factor plays a key role by increasing glomerular barrier permeability and causing podocyte injury. The presence of such factor is further supported by the fact, that primary FSGS has high recurrence rate after KT—up to 50% after the first KT and up to 100% in repeated transplantations [10]. Though the molecule has not been definitely identified, a considerable research has been performed in order to evaluate the role of TA in the treatment of FSGS.

TA is regarded in the treatment of primary FSGS only after treatment with steroids and calcineurin inhibitors (CNI) have failed. However, PEX/IA is considered as first-line treatment in recurrent FSGS after KT, as it leads to complete or partial remission in more than 50% of the KTRs [10]. They usually combined with immunosuppression—high-dose steroids, cyclophosphamide, higher doses of CNI and RTX. The needed number of procedures to achieve effective control of the disease by evaluating proteinuria is highly variable.

In recurrent FSGS PEX/IA are performed daily/every other day. The treatment should be started as early as possible in order to avoid progression of the disease. Proteinuria is the only marker that is used to assess the effect from the treatment. Treatment may have longer duration in order to avoid new episodes. Unfortunately, no predictors for TA effectivity in recurrent FSGS exist [10]. In addition, pre-transplant treatment failed to prevent recurrence of the disease [37].

Lipoprotein apheresis (LA) was assessed as a third TA modality in the treatment of FSGS. In LA lipoprotein particles are selectively removed from blood. The possible explanation for the benefit of this method is reducing the lipotoxic effect of hypercholesterolemia on podocyte function. Usually it is performed twice per week for 3 up to 6 weeks [10]. Currently LA is approved for primary/recurrent FSGS only in the USA.

3.2.2 Immunoglobulin A (IgA) nephropathy/Henoch-Schönlein Purpura

IgA nephropathy recurrence rate varies between 9 and 53% and is associated with poorer graft survival. Different predictors have been identified: crescentic forms of the disease, earlier onset of the primary disease, serum IgA levels, and steroid withdrawal after KT [38].

PEX did not prove to be effective in the treatment of primary IgA nephropathy [10, 39]. Indeed, predominantly cases with rapidly progressive crescentic IgA were evaluated without significant beneficial effect. The data for PEX treatment after KT are insufficient; therefore TA is generally not prescribed in recurrent IgA nephropathy. Similarly to IgA nephropathy, TA has no significant efficacy in Henoch-Schönlein Purpura.

3.2.3 Recurrent membranous nephropathy (MN)

Primary (idiopathic) membranous nephropathy (IMN) is characterized with the presence of autoantibodies against the podocyte localized phospholipase A2 receptor (anti-PLA2R). Currently, the recognized treatment options are cycling regimen (steroids/alkylating agent), CNI, or RTX. A single study demonstrated significant improvement from the combination of PEX + IVIG + RTX in resistant to conservative treatment (steroids/cyclophosphamide *or* CNI *or* RTX) IMN [40]. In this study, four PEX procedures were performed, coupled with a dose of 20 g IVIG and single dose RTX 375 mg/m^2.

The recurrence rate of IMN reaches 50%. High titers of anti-PLA2R were found to be a risk factor for recurrence after KT. Generally, switching from mTOR inhibitor to CNI is recommended, as well as use of RTX; alkylating agent should be avoided due to the risk for too potent immunosuppression [41]. Unfortunately, the role of TA in recurrent IMN is unclear and further research in this sphere is needed.

3.2.4 Recurrent membranoproliferative glomerulonephritis (MPGN)

Primary MPGN has two major types according to its pathogenesis: immune complex mediated and complement mediated. The new classification enables not only the better understanding of the disease, but also evaluates better the risk for recurrence after KT.

Immune complex-mediated MPGN is characterized by the glomerular deposition of polyclonal or monoclonal immunoglobulins. It is believed that the types and patterns of immunoglobulins may influence post-transplant characteristics of recurrent MPGN. For instance, IgG3k and IgG3λ deposits are linked to earlier recurrence and faster graft loss [41].

In the complex-mediated MPGN there are C3 glomerular deposits without immunoglobulin ones. It is known also as C3 glomerulopathy and consists of two entities—C3 glomerulonephritits and dense deposits disease (DDD). The two diseases have similar pathogenesis and clinical course. A recurrence rate up to 67% was reported for both diseases; DDD tended to recur later after KT and in both types graft failure was 50% [41, 42].

The suggested treatment so far includes PEX and immunosuppression—cyclophosphamide, RTX or eculizumab. However, the published studies are small and the results are inconsistent. Therefore larger trials are needed to evaluate the effectiveness of TA and the concomitant immunosuppressive agents in post-transplant MPGN [41].

3.2.5 Complement-mediated thrombotic microangiopathy (cmTMA, atypical hemolytic uremic syndrome)

Complement-mediated thrombotic microangiopathy (cmTMA), previously known as atypical hemolytic uremic syndrome is a life-threatening condition, which is caused by over-activation of the alternative pathway of the complement system. It presents with thrombocytopenia, microangiopathic hemolytic anemia, acute kidney injury, minimal to absent neurologic involvement, and fever. Over-activation is caused by genetic mutations causing impaired function of the alternative pathway inhibitors (factor H, membrane cofactor protein, and factor I) or overexpression of activators (factor B and complement component C3). Anti-Factor H autoantibodies can also cause cmTMA.

Generally, the disease's recurrence rate peaks up to 75% and is a significant predictor for poorer graft survival—90% of these grafts are lost within the first post-transplant year as the pathogenic serum proteins persist after the operation. However, membrane cofactor protein-associated cmTMA recurs significantly less—up to 20% after KT, with better graft survival due to the normal graft membrane proteins [43].

Initially, cmTMA was treated with daily PEX and immunosuppression. The recommended substitution fluid was FFP or FFP/albumin. However, with the introduction of Eculizumab in the treatment of the disease, the role of PEX is uncertain, as studies failed to demonstrate any advantage of PEX + Eculizumab vs. Eculizumab only [44]. PEX is reserved as first line therapy only in the presence of anti-Factor H autoantibodies, combined with immunosuppression [10].

3.2.6 Thrombotic thrombocytopenic purpura (TTP) after KT

TTP is TMA, characterized by similar clinical and laboratory findings as in cmTMA. However, it is more common in adults, presents with more pronounced thrombocytopenia, usually severe neurological impairment, and varying degree of renal insufficiency. In the post-transplant setting TTP is associated with CNI/mTOR inhibitors treatment, AbMR, viral infections, and ischemia reperfusion injury [45].

The key point in the treatment is correction of immunosuppressive treatment or treatment of the underlying condition. PEX can be included in the therapy, though the current data fail to demonstrate clear benefit from the procedure. Eculizumab proved to be more effective in these cases [46]. AbMR-associated TMA is usually treated with PEX + IVIG; RTX and Eculizumab can also be added to the treatment, especially in resistant to the standard PEX treatment cases [47, 48].

3.2.7 ANCA-associated vasculitis

The recurrence rate of ANCA-associated vasculitis is relatively low—approx. 10%. In these cases treatment as per general population is recommended.

Usually PEX is used in ANCA vasculitis in the native kidney in cases of rapidly deteriorating kidney function, diffuse alveolar hemorrhage, and serum creatinine above 5.7 mg/dl (504 μmol/L) [10, 39]. In recurrent ANCA vasculitis after KT the indications for TA are similar, usually the procedures are combined with immunosuppressive agents—steroids + cyclophosphamide or steroids + RTX [49]. Generally 7–12 procedures are needed. In alveolar hemorrhage the substitution fluid for PEX is FFP in order to avoid further increase in bleeding [10].

It is recommended in patients with ANCA vasculitis and end-stage renal disease transplantation to be delayed until a complete extrarenal remission for at least 12 months is achieved. However, ANCA-positive patients with extrarenal remission can be transplanted [39].

3.2.8 Recurrent/de novo anti-glomerular basement membrane (GBM) disease

Anti-GBM disease is usually caused by autoantibodies against the α3 chain of type IV collagen. The disease recurs in up to 50% of the cases post-transplant; the presence of detectable auto-antibodies' titer prior to KT is a well-established factor for recurrence. Therefore a period of at least 6 months of undetectable anti-GBM antibodies is recommended prior to KT [39].

De novo anti-GBM disease post-transplant usually develops in cases with Alport syndrome. In this clinical setting, the patients have impaired synthesis of collagen 4, with missing chains from α3 to α5 (usually α5), due to genetic mutations. After successful KT the graft expresses the normal α chains, which can trigger immunological response against these normal structures. De novo anti-GBM disease is detected in approx. 15% of the Alport patients after KT [7].

De novo anti-GBM disease presents with the symptoms of the disease in native kidneys. However, the recurrent form can present with subclinical course [50].

Generally, treatment is performed as per native kidneys' anti-GBM disease. Therapy should be initiated as early as possible. PEX is performed daily or every other day, anti-GBM antibody titers should be monitored and the procedure should be performed until the autoantibodies are undetectable (approx. 10–14 sessions). PEX is combined with steroids and cyclophosphamide; the role of RTX is currently unclear [10, 39].

3.2.9 Catastrophic antiphospholipid syndrome (cAPS)

Catastrophic antiphospholipid syndrome (cAPS) is acute life-threatening condition, associated with multiple thromboses in at least three systems within days or weeks, due to the presence of antiphospholipid antibodies (lupus anticoagulant, anticardiolipin, and anti-β2-glycoprotein I). The presence of cAPS is an indication for PEX. The procedure should be performed in combination with steroids ± IVIG and anticoagulants. This triple combination proved to be effective in cAPS. However, cyclophosphamide, eculizumab, and RTX were also used in the treatment [51]. PEX in cAPS is performed daily or every other day, substitution fluid is usually FFP or FFP + albumin [10].

The data for cAPS after KT are limited. The presence of antiphospholipid antibodies is a recognized risk factor for cAPS and anti-phospholipid syndrome (APS) recurrence [7]. A paper demonstrated that the use of Eculizumab can prevent post-transplant cAPS [52]. Barbour et al. demonstrated partial graft function improvement in patient with post-transplant cAPS, treated with PEX (28 procedures over 49 days), IVIG, and anticoagulation [53]. Further research in the field is needed, as the number of patients with APS/cAPS is small, especially those after KT.

4. Conclusions

TA has a well-established role in desensitization protocols prior to KT and treatment of AbMR in the post-transplant period. However, its place in the treatment of recurrent/de novo post-transplant glomerular disease is not fully understood due to the relatively small number of patients, insufficient controlled clinical trials, and different immunosuppressive agents used alongside with the procedure. In addition, the different TA modalities further complicate the assessment of TA effectivity. A multicenter approach could give better insight into TA role after renal transplantation and optimize its use in everyday clinical practice.

Author details

Jean Jeanov Filipov[1,2*] and Emil Paskalev Dimitrov[1,2]

1 Department of Nephrology and Transplantation, University Hospital "Alexandrovska", Sofia, Bulgaria

2 Medical University – Sofia, Sofia, Bulgaria

*Address all correspondence to: jeanphillipov@yahoo.com

References

[1] Garcia GG, Harden P, Chapman J. The global role of kidney transplantation. Kidney & Blood Pressure Research. 2012;**35**(5):299-304

[2] Otten HG, Verhaar MC, Borst HPE, Hené RJ, Zuilen ADV. Pretransplant donor-specific HLA class-I and -II antibodies are associated with an increased risk for kidney graft failure. American Journal of Transplantation. 2012;**12**(6):1618-1623

[3] Jung HY, Kim SH, Seo MY, Cho SY, Yang Y, Choi JY, et al. Characteristics and clinical significance of de novo donor-specific anti-HLA antibodies after kidney transplantation. Journal of Korean Medical Science. 2018;**33**(34):e217

[4] Agishi T, Kaneko I, Hasuo Y, Hayasaka Y, Sanaka T, Ota K, et al. Double filtration plasmapheresis. Therapeutic Apheresis. 2000;**4**(1): 29-33

[5] Kawamura A, Osanai M, Yonekawa M. Immunomodulation in transplant patients by cryofiltration. Therapeutic Apheresis. 1998;**2**(3):205-209

[6] Higgins R, Krishnan N, Hamer R, Fletcher S, Lam FT, Kashi H, et al. Renal transplantation across HLA antibodies as a successful treatment for dialysis hypotension syndrome; use of cryofiltration. Journal of Transplantation. 2010;**90**:948

[7] Salvadori M, Tsalouchos A. Therapeutic apheresis in kidney transplantation: An updated review. World Journal of Transplantation. 2019;**9**(6):103-122

[8] Samtleben W, Blumenstein M, RGH H. Indikationem zum Einsatz der Plasmapherese. MMW. 1982;**124**(27):641-645

[9] Grenda R, Durlik M. Eculizumab in renal transplantation: A 2017 update. Annals of Transplantation. 2017;**22**:550-554

[10] Padmanabhan A, Connelly-Smith L, Aqui N, Balogun RA, Klingel R, Meyer E, et al. Guidelines on the use of therapeutic apheresis in clinical practice - evidence-based approach from the writing Committee of the American Society for apheresis: The eighth special issue. Journal of Clinical Apheresis. 2019;**34**(3):171-354

[11] Morath C, Zeier M, Döhler B, Opelz G, Süsal C. ABO-incompatible kidney. Frontiers in Immunology. 2017;**8**:1-7

[12] Tydén G, Kumlien G, Genberg H, Sandberg J, Lundgren T, Fehrman I. ABO incompatible kidney transplantations without splenectomy, using antigen-specific immunoadsorption and rituximab. American Journal of Transplantation. 2005;**5**(1):145-148

[13] Ray DS, Thukral S. Outcome of ABO-incompatible living donor renal transplantations: A single-center experience from eastern India. Transplantation Proceedings. 2016;**48**(8):2622-2628

[14] Jha PK, Tiwari AK, Bansal SB, Sethi SK, Ahlawat R, Kher V. Cascade plasmapheresis as preconditioning regimen for ABO-incompatible renal transplantation: A single-center experience. Transfusion. 2016;**56**(4):956-961

[15] Hiesse C, Kriaa F, Rousseau P, Farahmand H, Bismuth A, Fries D, et al. Immunoadsorption of anti-hla antibodies for highly sensitized patients awaiting renal transplantation. Nephrology, Dialysis, Transplantation. 1992;**7**(9):944-951

[16] Alarabi A, Backman U, Wikström B, Sjöberg O, Tufveson G. Plasmapheresis in HLA-immunosensitized patients prior to kidney transplantation. The International Journal of Artificial Organs. 1997;**20**(1):51-56

[17] Morath C, Beimler J, Opelz G, Ovens J, Scherer S, Schwenger V, et al. An integrative approach for the transplantation of high-risk sensitized patients. Transplantationsmedizin: Organ der Deutschen Transplantationsgesellschaft. 2009;**21**(Suppl. 2):128-129

[18] Loupy A, Suberbielle-Boissel C, Zuber J, Anglicheau D, Timsit MO, Martinez F, et al. Combined posttransplant prophylactic IVIg/anti-CD 20/plasmapheresis in kidney recipients with preformed donor-specific antibodies: A pilot study. Transplantation. 2010;**89**(11):1403-1410

[19] Amrouche L, Aubert O, Suberbielle C, Rabant M, Van Huyen JPD, Martinez F, et al. Long-term outcomes of kidney transplantation in patients with high levels of preformed DSA: The Necker high-risk transplant program. Transplantation. 2017;**101**(10):2440-2448

[20] Bartel G, Wahrmann M, Regele H, Kikić Ž, Fischer G, Druml W, et al. Peritransplant immunoadsorption for positive crossmatch deceased donor kidney transplantation. American Journal of Transplantation. 2010;**10**(9):2033-2042

[21] Schwaiger E, Eskandary F, Kozakowski N, Bond G, Ẑeljko K, Yoo D, et al. Deceased donor kidney transplantation across donor-specific antibody barriers: Predictors of antibody-mediated rejection. Nephrology, Dialysis, Transplantation. 2016;**31**(8):1342-1351

[22] Orandi BJ, Luo X, Massie AB, Garonzik-Wang JM, Lonze BE, Ahmed R, et al. Survival benefit with kidney transplants from HLA-incompatible live donors. The New England Journal of Medicine. 2016;**374**(10):940-950

[23] Montgomery RA, Lonze BE, King KE, Kraus ES, Kucirka LM, Locke JE, et al. Desensitization in HLA-incompatible kidney recipients and survival. The New England Journal of Medicine. 2011;**365**(4):318-326

[24] Thielke JJ, West-Thielke PM, Herren HL, Bareato U, Ommert T, Vidanovic V, et al. Living donor kidney transplantation across positive crossmatch: The University of Illinois at Chicago experience. Transplantation. 2009;**87**(2):268-273

[25] Klein K, Süsal C, Schäfer SM, Becker LE, Beimler J, Schwenger V, et al. Living donor kidney transplantation in patients with donor-specific HLA antibodies enabled by anti-CD20 therapy and peritransplant apheresis. Atherosclerosis. Supplements. 2013;**14**(1):199-202

[26] Rostaing L, Congy N, Allal A, Esposito L, Sallusto F, Doumerc N, et al. Successful transplantation in ABO-and HLA-incompatible kidney-transplant patients. Transplant International. 2016;**29**:16

[27] Wiseman AC. Prophylaxis and treatment of kidney transplant rejection. In: Floege J, Johnson RJFJ, editors. Comprehensive Clinical Nephrology. 4th ed. St Louis: Elsevier Saunders; 2010. pp. 1166-1176

[28] Haas M, Sis B, Racusen LC, Solez K, Glotz D, Colvin RB, et al. Banff 2013 meeting report: Inclusion of C4d-negative antibody-mediated rejection and antibody-associated arterial lesions. American Journal of Transplantation. 2014;**14**(2):272-283

[29] Lefaucheur C, Loupy A, Vernerey D, Duong-Van-Huyen JP, Suberbielle C,

Anglicheau D, et al. Antibody-mediated vascular rejection of kidney allografts: A population-based study. Lancet. 2013;**381**(9863):313-319

[30] Bailly E, Blancho G, Ville S, Morelon E, Bamoulid J, Caillard S, et al. Five-year outcomes after randomized treatment by rituximab in early acute antibody-mediated rejection in renal transplantation: Long term outcomes of the RITUX ERAH study. American Journal of Transplantation. 2018;**18**(Supplement 4):253

[31] Wan SS, Ying TD, Wyburn K, Roberts DM, Wyld M, Chadban SJ. The treatment of antibody-mediated rejection in kidney transplantation: An updated systematic review and meta-analysis. Transplantation. 2018;**102**(4):557-568

[32] Tan J, Stéphan B, Scandling JD. Clinical management. In: Taal M, Certow BB, et al., editors. The Kidney. 9th ed. Philadelphia: Elsevier Saunders; 2012. pp. 2515-2551

[33] Campos ÉF, Tedesco-Silva H, Machado PG, Franco M, Medina-Pestana JO, Gerbase-DeLima M. Post-transplant anti-HLA class II antibodies as risk factor for late kidney allograft failure. American Journal of Transplantation. 2006;**6**(10):2316-2320

[34] Yamamoto T, Watarai Y, Takeda A, Tsujita M, Hiramitsu T, Goto N, et al. De novo anti-HLA DSA characteristics and subclinical antibody-mediated kidney allograft injury. Transplantation. 2016;**100**(10):2194-2202

[35] Susal C, Wettstein D, Dohler B, Morath C, Ruhenstroth A, Scherer S, et al. Association of Kidney Graft Loss with de novo produced donor-specific and non-donor-specific HLA antibodies detected by single antigen testing. Transplantation. 2015;**99**(9):1976-1980

[36] Krum K, Fagoga O, Doshi M. Role of non-donor specific HLA antibodies (NDSA) in kidney transplant rejection. Transplantation. 2014;**98**:435

[37] Verghese PS, Rheault MN, Jackson S, Matas AJ, Chinnakotla S, Chavers B. The effect of peri-transplant plasmapheresis in the prevention of recurrent FSGS. Pediatric Transplantation. 2018;**22**(3):e13154. DOI: 10.1111/petr.13154

[38] Moroni G, Belingheri M, Frontini G, Tamborini F, Messa P. Immunoglobulin a nephropathy. Recurrence after renal transplantation. Frontiers in Immunology. 2019;**10**:1332

[39] Kidney Disease: Improving Global Outcomes (KDIGO) Glomerulonephritis Work Group. KDIGO clinical practice guideline for glomerulonephritis. Kidney International. Supplement. 2012;**2**(2):139-274

[40] Müller-Deile J, Schiffer L, Hiss M, Haller H, Schiffer M. A new rescue regimen with plasma exchange and rituximab in high-risk membranous glomerulonephritis. European Journal of Clinical Investigation. 2015;**45**(12):1260-1269

[41] Lim WH, Shingde M, Wong G. Recurrent and de novo glomerulonephritis after kidney transplantation. Frontiers in Immunology. 2019;**10**:1944

[42] Zand L, Lorenz EC, Cosio FG, Fervenza FC, Nasr SH, Gandhi MJ, et al. Clinical findings, pathology, and outcomes of C3GN after kidney transplantation. Journal of the American Society of Nephrology. 2014;**25**(5):1110-1117

[43] Sellier-Leclerc AL, Fremeaux-Bacchi V, Dragon-Durey MA, Macher MA, Niaudet P, Guest G, et al. Differential impact of complement mutations on clinical characteristics in atypical hemolytic uremic syndrome. Journal of the American Society of Nephrology. 2007;**18**(8):2392-2400

[44] Krishnappa V, Gupta M, Elrifai M, Moftakhar B, Ensley MJ, Vachharajani TJ, et al. Atypical hemolytic uremic syndrome: A meta-analysis of case reports confirms the prevalence of genetic mutations and the shift of treatment regimens. Therapeutic Apheresis and Dialysis. 2018;**22**(2):178-188

[45] Abbas F, El Kossi M, Kim JJ, Sharma A, Halawa A. Thrombotic microangiopathy after renal transplantation: Current insights in de novo and recurrent disease. World Journal of Transplantation. 2018;**8**(5):122-141

[46] Epperla N, Hemauer K, Hamadani M, Friedman KD, Kreuziger LB. Impact of treatment and outcomes for patients with posttransplant drug-associated thrombotic microangiopathy. Transfusion. 2017;**57**(11):2775-2781

[47] Satoskar AA, Pelletier R, Adams P, Nadasdy GM, Brodsky S, Pesavento T, et al. De novo thrombotic microangiopathy in renal allograft biopsies - role of antibody-mediated rejection. American Journal of Transplantation. 2010;**10**(8):1804-1811

[48] Garg N, Rennke HG, Pavlakis M, Zandi-Nejad K. De novo thrombotic microangiopathy after kidney transplantation. Transplantation Reviews. 2018;**32**(1):58-68

[49] Walters G. Role of therapeutic plasmapheresis in ANCA-associated vasculitis. Pediatric Nephrology. 2016;**31**(2):217-225

[50] Kotanko P, Pusey CD, Levy JB. Recurrent glomerulonephritis following renal transplantation. Transplantation. 1997;**63**(8):1045-1052

[51] Cervera R, Rodríguez-Pintó I, Espinosa G. The diagnosis and clinical management of the catastrophic antiphospholipid syndrome: A comprehensive review. Journal of Autoimmunity. 2018;**92**:1-11

[52] Lonze BE, Zachary AA, Magro CM, Desai NM, Orandi BJ, Dagher NN, et al. Eculizumab prevents recurrent antiphospholipid antibody syndrome and enables successful renal transplantation. American Journal of Transplantation. 2014;**14**(2):459-465

[53] Barbour TD, Crosthwaite A, Chow K, Finlay MJ, Better N, Hughes PD, et al. Antiphospholipid syndrome in renal transplantation. Nephrology. 2014;**19**(4):177-185

Section 3

New Features of the Host-Pathogen Relationship

Chapter 5

Bacterial Resistance in Urinary Tract Infections: Multidrug Resistant ESBL Producing Gram Negative Uropathogens from Patients

Akosua Bonsu Karikari, Courage Kosi Setsoafia Saba and David Yembilla Yamik

Abstract

Urinary tract infection is one of the most common bacterial infectious diseases encountered in clinical practice. The development and spread of multidrug resistant isolates are of great global health burden; among them, extended spectrum beta-lactamase (ESBL) producing Enterobacteriaceae has been a prime concern. This topic describes the resistance patterns of eighty three (83) Gram negative uropathogens to different classes of antibiotics. Bacteria isolates were obtained from patients of all age groups who sought medical attention at a secondary and tertiary hospital in Northern Ghana. Culture and isolation methods employed were the quantitative urine culture on Cysteine Lysine Electrolyte Deficient (CLED) agar and standard biochemical tests. ESBL production was detected using the CLSI recommended phenotypic confirmatory test along with routine antibiotic susceptibility test, adopting the Kirby-Bauer disk diffusion method. Out of 83 isolates, seven (7) Gram negative uropathogens were characterized and ESBLs were detected in 32 of the isolates. *Escherichia coli* was the pathogen with most ESBL positive strains. Generally high and multiple drug resistance were recorded in both ESBL and non-ESBL strains to the empirical drugs, however, ESBL positive strains significantly ($p = 0.000$) showed greater resistance. A notable finding was the appreciable resistance exhibited by ESBL strains to last line treatment drugs that include aminoglycosides and imipenem.

Keywords: Antibiotic resistance, ESBLs, Gram negative uropathogens, UTI, Ghana

1. Introduction

Urinary tract infection (UTI) is a disease of the genitourinary tract that is common in all gender and age groups. Bacteria are the major cause responsible for more than 95% of UTI cases. *Escherichia coli* is the most prevalent causative organism and solely accounts for more than 80% of the infections [1].

In recent times multiple drug resistance among bacteria uropathogens has significantly increased mainly due to the spread of extended spectrum β-lactamases (ESBLs). ESBLs are the enzymes, mostly encoded by plasmids in effect of mutation due to which bacteria show resistance to various β-lactam antibiotics including cephalosporins and monobactams [2]. More than one hundred and fifty (150) ESBL types have been identified and majority of them belong to *class A* enzymes SHV, TEM and CTX-M [3]. These *class A* enzymes hydrolyse penicillin, oxyimino-cephalosporins, and monobactams but not carbapenems or cephamycins and are inhibited *in vitro* by clavulanate [4]. There is a growing apprehension for multidrug-resistant Gram-negative bacteria which produce extended-spectrum β-lactamases [5, 6]. Members of the *Enterobacteriaceae* primarily produce ESBLs particularly *Klebsiella pneumoniae, K. oxytoca* and *E. coli*, then again, other Gram-negative organisms including *Salmonella*, *Pseudomonas aeruginosa*, *Proteus spp.* and *Acinetobacter baumannii* have also been named [7].

Immunosuppressed patients with invasive devices, prolonged hospital admissions and long term antibiotic exposure are predisposing factors for colonization or infection with ESBL pathogens [8]. Detecting ESBL producers is a major challenge in clinical settings because of selective pressure caused by heavy use of expanded-spectrum cephalosporins and failures in effective infection control measures in hospitals [9]. Delayed reporting of ESBL producing Gram-negative bacilli is associated with extended clinical admission, increased morbidity and mortality as well as high health care expenditures [4].

Several tests have been recommended for detection of ESBL production *in vitro.* The most frequently used methods include double disc synergy test, combined disc method and E-test. Many automated systems have also been developed for diagnosis while some laboratories use molecular methods for establishing ESBL phenomenon [10].

Still lacking in several healthcare facilities in developing countries including Ghana are laboratories for urine culture and antimicrobial susceptibility testing which obviously lead to unavailable data on ESBLs. Records of prevailing levels of antimicrobial resistance among pathogens are valuable in taking appropriate empirical therapy decisions. Local data of pathogens' susceptibility to antibiotics is virtually absent in most hospitals in Northern Ghana. The purpose of this study was to characterize and screen Gram-negative uropathogens to detect ESBL producers and determine the susceptibility pattern of strains from patients in a secondary and tertiary care hospitals in Northern Ghana. Authors report on the incidence of ESBL-positive Gram negative bacilli in patients presenting with UTI infections in Northern Ghana.

2. Materials and methods

Data was prospectively collected for a period of six (6) months (April 2018 to September 2018) at a tertiary and secondary care hospital in the Northern region of Ghana. A total of 738 non-repetitive mid-stream urine samples were cultured on Cysteine Lysine Electrolyte Deficient Medium (CLED) and isolates were identified by standard laboratory methods [11]. Strains totaling one hundred and ninety (190) were identified and considered clinically relevant which consisted of 107 Gram positives and 83 Gram negative bacilli. In assessing the prevalence of ESBL production among the Gram negative uropathogens, all 83 isolates were further processed for ESBL detection.

Antimicrobial susceptibility was determined by the Kirby-Bauer disc diffusion method according to Clinical Laboratory Standard Institute (CLSI) guidelines [12].

The drugs used for antibiogram determination were imipenem (10 μg), norfloxacin (10 μg) nitrofurantoin (50 μg), amikacin (30 μg), gentamicin (10 μg), trimethoprim–sulphamethoxazole (co-trimoxazole) (25 μg), ampicillin (10 μg), chloramphenicol (30 μg), tetracycline (30 μg), ceftriaxone (30 μg), cefoxitin (30 μg), ciprofloxacin (10 μg), augmentin (30 μg), and erythromycin (15 μg). Culture media and all antibiotic discs were sourced from Oxoid. Multiple drug resistance was defined as resistance to three (3) or more classes of antibiotics.

ESBL production was detected by using the CLSI recommended phenotypic confirmatory test along with routine antibiotic susceptibility testing. This was performed with ceftadizime (CAZ 30 μg) and cefotaxime (CTX 30 μg) discs alone and in combination with clavulanic acid (CAZ/CLA 30/10 μg). A ≥ 5 mm increase in zone size of the combined ceftazidime and clavulanic acid was considered as confirmation of ESBL production [12]. All the recovered Gram negative bacteria were subjected to ESBL screening although CLSI phenotypic confirmatory test endorses *Escherichia coli*, *Klebsiella pneumoniae* and *Proteus mirabilis*. *Escherichia coli* ATCC 25922 was used as negative control for ESBL production due to unavailability of a positive control strain. All susceptibility testing was performed on Mueller-Hinton agar using 0.5 McFarland suspension from overnight cultures, followed by incubation at 35°C for 16 to 18 hrs.

SPSS version 20 was used to analyze the data. Descriptive statistics including frequencies and percentages were used. Pearson chi-square test at 95% significant level was conducted to determine associations between categorical outcome variables. A two tailed p-value of <0.05 was considered statistically significant. Approval for the study was obtained from the Ethical Review Committee of the Tamale Teaching Hospital.

3. Results

Out of the 738 urine screened, 190 were considered significant bacteuria. The 190 uropathogens comprised 107 Gram positives and 83 Gram negatives. Of the 83 Gram negative isolates screened, 32 (38.6%) were positive for ESBL production and *E. coli* was the predominant (37.5%) ESBL producing pathogen. About 81% (26) of the ESBL strains came from in-patients and approximately 38% were recovered from patients who were 60 years and above. ESBL-positive strains were significantly (P = 0.002) greater in female isolates (**Table 1**).

	No. ESBL positive patients	Percentage (%)	P-value
Age			
< 20	2	6.3	0.000
20–39	11	34.4	
40–59	7	21.4	
60 and Above	12	37.5	
Sex			
Male	15	46.9	0.002
Female	17	53.1	
Total	32	100.0	

Table 1.
Gender and age distribution of patients with ESBL positive strains.

Comparing ESBL and non-ESBL strains, the difference in resistance pattern was significant, p = 0.000. ESBL producing strains showed up to 50% resistance to aminoglycosides (gentamicin and amikacin) and about 22% to imipenem while resistance of non-ESBLs were below 10% to aminoglycosides (gentamicin and amikacin) and approximately 10% to imipenem. The non-ESBL strains were highly resistant (70–90%) to only ampicillin, erythromycin, nitrofurantoin and tetracycline but ESBL strains generally showed high resistance (50–100%) to almost all the drugs, with exception to amikacin and imipenem where resistance was below 30%. Resistance to cefepime was about 84% among ESBL strains and 19.6% in the non-ESBL strains (**Table 2**).

Multidrug resistance was a common occurrence in the ESBL strains with approximately 68% of them being resistant to six (6) or more antibiotics but only 15.7% of the non-ESBL strains showed this particular phenomenon, **Table 3**. All ESBL positive and negative strains of *E. coli*, *Klebsiella* and *Salmonella* showed 100% multiple drug resistance (**Table 4**).

Resistance of β-lactamase producing *E. coli* strains to the quinolones (ciprofloxacin, norfloxacin) were up to 83%, however the non- β-lactamase producing strains showed resistance of about 26–30% to the same class of drugs. Also, against the 3rd generation cephalosporins (ceftriaxone, ceftazidime and cefotaxime) the β-lactamase producers showed resistance of 83–100%, but resistance was between 21 and 26% among the non- β-lactamase *E. coli* strains (**Table 5**).

Klebsiella strains that were β-lactamase positive showed resistance of up to 44% to the quinolones while strains that did not produce β-lactamase had resistance of about 33%. Resistance to the aminoglycosides were 22–66.7% in the ESBL strains and 0% in the non-ESBL strains. Against the 3rd generation cephalosporins, the ESBL strains showed resistance of 88–100% as the non-ESBL strains had resistance of 16–33% (**Table 5**).

Antibiotic	% ESBL Strains (n = 32)	% Non-ESBL Strains (n = 51)	P-Value
Cefoxitin	53.1	39.2	0.000
cefepime	84.4	19.6	
Ciprofloxacin	59.4	21.6	
Norfloxacin	62.5	23.5	
Amikacin	21.9	7.8	
Gentamicin	50.0	7.8	
Ampicillin	96.9	90.2	
Augmentin	62.5	31.4	
Tetracycline	78.1	70.6	
Ceftriaxone	84.4	23.5	
Ceftazidime	93.8	27.5	
Nitrofurantoin	75.0	72.5	
Chloramphenicol	59.4	54.9	
Erythromycin	75.0	86.3	
Cotrimoxazole	78.1	64.7	
Imipenem	21.9	9.8	
Cefotaxime	100.0	31.4	

Table 2.
Resistance pattern of ESBL and non ESBL strains of UTI patients.

Multidrug Resistance	ESBL Producers	Non ESBL Producers	P-Value
	No. of Resistant Strains (%)	No. of Resistant Strains (%)	
3 Classes of antibiotics	3(9.7)	27(52.9)	0.000
4 Classes of antibiotics	2(6.5)	12(23.5)	
5 Classes of antibiotics	5(16.1)	4(7.8)	
6 Classes of antibiotics	7(22.6)	2(3.9)	
≥7 Classes of antibiotics	14(45.2)	6(11.8)	
Total	31(100.0)	51(100.0)	

Table 3.
Multidrug resistance of ESBL and non ESBL strains.

Organism	ESBL Producers		Non- ESBL Producers		P -Value
	Isolates (n)	MDR (%)	Isolates	MDR (%)	
E.coli	12	12(100.0)	23	23(100.0)	0.204
Salmonella	2	2(100.0)	2	2(100.0)	
Klebsiella	9	9(100.0)	6	6(100.0)	
Enterobacter	4	4(100.0)	12	12(100.0)	
Serratia	4	3(75.0)	7	7(100.0)	
Pseudomonas	0	0(0.0)	1	1(100.0	
Proteus	1	1(100.0)	0	0(0.0)	

Table 4.
Multidrug resistance rate of uropathogens.

Enterobacter producing ESBL showed 75% resistance to the quinolones while 0% resistance was observed in the non-ESBL strains and to the aminoglycosides resistance were 25–50% in the ESBL strains and 0% among the non-ESBL strains (**Table 5**).

ESBL-positive *E. coli, Klebsiella* and *Enterobacter*, showed respective resistivity of 25%. 33.3% and 25% to Imipenem while in the non-ESBL strains, resistance were 8.7% in *E. coli* and 0% each in *Klebsiella* and *Enterobacter* sp. (**Table 5**).

4. Discussion

In recent times antimicrobial resistance has been acknowledged as a major public health problem worldwide with developing countries reporting more worrying trends. The emergence and rapid dissemination of multiple drug resistant pathogens including ESBL producing Enterobacteriaceae have made management of hospital and community acquired infections caused by these strains difficult. The prevalence of ESBL producing pathogens greatly differs from country to country and also within country. Prevalence ranging from below 1% to more than 70% have been documented globally [13].

We identified seven (7) species of Gram negative uropathogens and detected ESBLs in 32 (38.6%) out of 83 uropathogens recovered from patients reporting to hospitals in Northern Ghana. Among the Seven (7) Gram negative species screened for ESBL production, *E. coli* was the pathogen with the most (37.5%) ESBL positive strains which is comparable to reported rates from India [14], Turkey [15]

Organism	Antibiotics																
	FOX	FEP	CIP	NOR	AK	GEN	AMP	ACA	TE	CRO	CAZ	NIT	CHL	ERY	COT	IPM	CTX
ESBL strains																	
E. coli (12)	33.3	91.7	83.3	83.3	25.0	41.7	100.0	58.3	100.0	83.3	100.0	66.7	50.0	75.0	91.7	25.0	100.0
Salmonella (2)	100.0	50.0	0.0	0.0	0.0	100.0	100.0	50.0	50.0	100.0	100.0	100.0	100.0	100.0	50.0	0.0	100.0
Klebsiella (9)	77.8	77.8	44.4	33.3	22.2	66.7	100.0	66.7	55.6	88.9	88.9	88.9	77.8	77.8	66.7	33.3	100.0
Enterobacter (4)	75.0	100.0	75.0	75.0	25.0	50.0	100.0	75.0	100.0	100.0	100.0	50.0	25.0	100.0	100.0	25.0	100.0
Serratia (4)	25.0	100.0	50.0	75.0	25.0	25.0	75.0	50.0	50.0	50.0	100.0	75.0	50.0	50.0	50.0	0.0	100.0
Proteus (1)	0.0	0.0	0.0	100	0.0	0.0	100.0	100.0	100.0	100.0	0.0	100.0	100.0	0.0	100.0	0.0	100.0
Non-ESBL strains																	
E.coli (23)	21.7	21.7	26.1	30.4	17.4	4.4	87.0	17.4	87.0	26.1	21.7	56.5	56.5	91.3	78.3	8.7	26.1
Salmonella (2)	100.0	0.0	100.0	100	0.0	100.0	100.0	100.0	100.0	100	100.0	100	100.0	100	100.0	50.0	100.0
Klebsiella (6)	50.0	16.7	33.3	33.3	0.0	0.0	100.0	50.0	66.7	33.3	33.3	66.7	50.0	83.3	83.3	0.0	16.7
*Enterobacte*r (12)	41.7	8.3	0.0	0.0	0.0	0.0	83.3	16.7	58.3	0.0	16.7	83.3	33.3	91.7	33.3	0.0	16.7
Serratia (7)	57.1	42.9	14.3	14.3	0.0	14.3	100.0	57.1	28.6	14.3	42.9	100.0	71.4	71.4	42.9	14.3	57.1
Pseudomonas (1)	100.0	0.0	0.0	0.0	0.0	0.0	100.0	100.0	100.0	100	0.0	100.0	100.0	0.0	100.0	100.0	100.0

FOX, Cefoxitin; FEP, Cefepime; CIP, Ciprofloxacin; NOR, Norfloxacin; AK, Amikacin; GN, Gentamycin; AMP, Ampicillin; ACA, Augmentin; TE, Tetracycline; CRO, Ceftriaxone; CAZ, Ceftazidime; NIT, Nitrofurantoin; CHL, Chloramphenicol; ERY, Erythromycin; COT, Co-trimoxazole; IPM, Imipenem; CTX, Cefotaxime.

Table 5.
Resistance pattern of non ESBL and ESBL producing uropathogens.

and Saudi Arabia [16], but lower than a report from Egypt [17]. Moreover, in Africa, the prevalence of ESBL- producing *E. coli* has been found to range from 35 to 65% [18]. From literature, ESBLs are produced primarily by members of the Enterobacteriaceae and other pathogens including *Acinetobacter baumannii, Proteus* spp., *Pseudomonas aeruginosa* and *Salmonella* spp. [19] but detection is more frequent in *E. coli* and *Klebsiella* species [20].

ESBL positivity was significant in females (0.002) compared to the male gender. In contrast, authors from India [14] and Israel [21] have reported male prevalence citing male gender as a risk factor for community-acquired ESBL-positive UTI [21]. Our study however involved in-patient and OPD cases of UTI with 81% of strains coming from in-patients, which possibly could account for the difference in results. Besides, females are often beset with UTI due to settlement of colonic Gram negative bacteria on the urethra as a consequence of a short urethra and its closeness to the anus. The gender of a patient, according to Magliano and colleagues is one of the risk factors of UTI [22].

Age group 60 and beyond (37.5%) were mostly found with ESBL positive strains. Several studies have indicated age over 60 years to be an associated risk factor for community-acquired infections with ESBL-producing microorganisms in adults [21, 23, 24]. This age bracket is putatively prone to infections, which is expected to make them consume antibiotics in greater quantities that could ultimately contribute to drug resistance.

Therapeutic challenge is allied with ESBL-producing strains due to low susceptibility to variety of β-lactams, including third generation cephalosporins as well as the possibility for plasmid mediated quinolone and carbapenem resistance. The ESBL isolates showed high rates of resistance to all studied antibiotics with exception to amikacin and imipenem, where resistance to these drugs were 21.9% each. The 21.9% may be considered high when compared to documented rates in different geographical regions where susceptibility to imipenem was 100% [13, 25, 26]. The resistant pattern of our study isolates reaffirms accounts of low susceptibility of ESBL strains to third generation cephalosporins and other β-lactam drugs. Respective resistances of ESBL strains to the third generation cephalosporins; cefotaxime, ceftazidime and ceftriaxone were 100%, 93.8% and 84.4% and 31.4%, 27.5% and 23.5% were for non-ESBL strains and the difference was statistically significant (0.000). Similarly, susceptibility of ESBL strains to ampicillin and augmentin were low (62.5–96.9% resistance). The non-ESBL strains however showed equally high resistance to ampicillin (90.2%) and rather lower resistance (31.4%) to augmentin.

Antibiotics including quinolones (ciprofloxacin, norfloxacin), cefepime, tetracycline, cotrimoxazole had ESBL positive strains exhibiting greater resistance to them as opposed to non-ESBL strains with a significant difference. Quite the reverse occurred with erythromycin where non-ESBL isolates resistance (86.3%) was significantly more than the ESBLs (75.0%); but almost equal resistance was observed in ESBLs (75.0%) and non-ESBL strains (72.5%) to nitrofurantoin.

A notable finding of this research was the high resistance of both ESBL and non-ESBL strains to first line and empirical drugs of UTI. Multiple drug resistance of 100% was observed in six (6) of the seven (7) uropathogens identified and close to 66% of the ESBL strains were resistant to six (6) or more antibiotics. Additionally, resistance to aminoglycosides which have reportedly been low [13, 27–29] and considered a treatment option for complicated UTI was not effective against our ESBL strains, with up to 50% of strains showing resistance. Limiting the use of a group of antibiotics could lead to over prescription of other classes resulting in a surge of resistance in the oversubscribed drugs. The rampant pathogen resistant reports to frequently used and affordable drugs are gradually putting pressure on the last line class of drugs including the carbapenems. A review of antimicrobial resistance studies in Ghana have shown a steady rise in resistance to classes of antibiotics such as aminoglycosides and carbapenems (personal review, unpublished) which previously were very effective and rarely suffered pathogen resistance. This research documented 21.9% resistance from ESBL strains and almost 10% from Non-ESBL isolates to imipenem. This clinical warning of increased resistance to last line antibiotics and high MDR records prompt an immediate need to formulate strategic policy initiatives to reduce their emergence and spread. Regulating the emergence and spread of ESBL organisms in hospitals require a blend of antimicrobial stewardship and effective infection control compliance in hospitals. Consistent monitoring of regional and national surveillance data of the common infectious pathogens besides screening of ESBL producers is of prime importance in controlling the rise in multi-drug resistant pathogens.

5. Conclusion

The study found *E. coli* with most ESBL producing strains. Multiple drug resistance was a common occurrence; in almost all the Gram negative uropathogens characterized, 100% resistance was recorded. ESBL strains generally showed greater resistance than the non-ESBL strains particularly to the cephalosporins and β-lactam antibiotics. However resistance to UTI empirical drugs and other commonly used antibiotics were alike in both ESBL and non-ESBL strains as low susceptibility was observed. An important finding was the considerable resistance of the ESBL strains to the aminoglycosides and imipenem which are last line treatment drugs. The results of the study clearly indicate the need for antimicrobial stewardship and enhanced infection control measures in our hospitals. Routine screening of ESBLs in our hospitals is highly recommended since appropriate antimicrobial therapy can only commence with early detection of these strains.

Author details

Akosua Bonsu Karikari[1]*, Courage Kosi Setsoafia Saba[2] and David Yembilla Yamik[3]

1 Department of Clinical Microbiology, School of Medicine and Health Sciences, University for Development Studies, Tamale, Ghana

2 Department of Microbiology, Faculty of Biosciences, University for Development Studies, Tamale, Ghana

3 Department of Biotechnology, Faculty of Biosciences, University for Development Studies, Tamale, Ghana

*Address all correspondence to: asbuks@yahoo.co.uk

References

[1] Nachimuthu R, Chettipalayam S, Velramar B, Kurumandur R, Velu R. Urinary tract infection and antimicrobial susceptibility pattern of extended spectrum beta lactamase producing clinical isolates. Adv Biol Res (Faisalabad) 2008; 2(5-6): 78-82.

[2] Ummadevi S, Joseph NM, Kumari K, Easow JM, Kumar S, Stephen S. Detection of ESBLs, AmpC beta lactamase and metallo-beta-lactamases in clinical isolates of ceftazidime resistant P. aeruginosa. BJM. 2011;42(1): 1284-1288.

[3] Mendelson G, Hait V, Ben-Israel J, Gronich D, Granot E, Raz R. Prevalence and risk factors of extended-spectrum beta-lactamase-producing *Escherichia coli* and *Klebsiella pneumoniae* in an Israeli long-term care facility. European Journal of Clinical Microbiology and Infectious Diseases. 2005;24(1):17-22.

[4] Mehrgan H, Rahbar M. Prevalence of extended-spectrum β-lactamase-producing *Escherichia coli* in a tertiary care hospital in Tehran, Iran. International journal of antimicrobial agents. 2008;31(2):147-151.

[5] Dhillon RH, Clark J. ESBLs: a clear and present danger?. Critical care research and practice. 2012;2012.

[6] World Health Organisation. WHO Publishes List of Bacteria for Which New Antibiotics are Urgently Needed. Available online: https://www.who.int/news-room/detail/27-02-2017-who-publishes-list-of-bacteria-for-which-newantibiotics-are-urgently-needed (accessed on 14 August 2020).

[7] Falagas ME, Karageorgopoulos DE. Extended-spectrum β-lactamase-producing organisms. Journal of Hospital infection. 2009;73(4): 345-354.

[8] Paterson DL, Bonomo RA. Extended-spectrum β-lactamases: a clinical update. Clinical microbiology reviews. 2005;18(4):657-686.

[9] Roopa TJ, Sudha SS. Antimicrobial susceptibility of extended spectrum beta–lactamase (ESBL) producing uropathogens isolated from ICU patients. International Journal of Biological Technology. 2010;1:23-31.

[10] Drieux L, Brossier F, Sougakoff W, Jarlier V. Phenotypic detection of extended-spectrum β-lactamase production in *Enterobacteriaceae*: review and bench guide. Clinical Microbiology and Infection. 2008;14:90-103.

[11] Versalovic J, Carroll KC, Funke G, Jorgensen JH, Landry ML, Warnock DW. Manual of clinical microbiology. 2011.

[12] Wayne PA. Clinical and laboratory standards institute. Performance standards for antimicrobial susceptibility testing. 2013.

[13] Shakya P, Shrestha D, Maharjan E, Sharma VK, Paudyal R. ESBL production among *E. coli* and *Klebsiella* spp. causing urinary tract infection: a hospital based study. The Open Microbiology Journal. 2017;11:23.

[14] Nisha KV, Veena SA, Rathika SD, Vijaya SM, Avinash SK. Antimicrobial susceptibility, risk factors and prevalence of bla cefotaximase, temoneira, and sulfhydryl variable genes among *Escherichia coli* in community-acquired pediatric urinary tract infection. Journal of Laboratory Physicians. 2017;9(3):156.

[15] Kizilca O, Siraneci R, Yilmaz A, Hatipoglu N, Ozturk E, Kiyak A, Ozkok D. Risk factors for community-acquired urinary tract infection caused by ESBL-producing bacteria in children.

Pediatrics International. 2012;54(6): 858-862.

[16] El-Kersh TA, Marie MA, Al-Sheikh YA, Al-Kahtani SA. Prevalence and risk factors of community-acquired urinary tract infections due to ESBL-producing Gram negative bacteria in an Armed Forces Hospital in Sothern Saudi Arabia. Global Advanced Research Journal of Medicine and Medical Science. 2015;4(7):321-330.

[17] Hassuna NA, Khairalla AS, Farahat EM, Hammad AM, Abdel-Fattah M. Molecular characterization of Extended-spectrum β lactamase-producing *E. coli* recovered from community-acquired urinary tract infections in Upper Egypt. Scientific Reports. 2020;10(1):1-8.

[18] Afunwa RA, Odimegwu DC, Iroha RI, Esimone CO. Antimicrobial resistance status and prevalence rates of extended spectrum beta-lactamase producers isolated from a mixed human population. Bosnian Journal of Basic Medical Sciences. 2011;11(2):91.

[19] Vandana KE, Honnavar P. AmpC beta lactamases among ESBL producing *Escherichia coli* and *Klebsiella pneumoniae*-If you don't look, you won't find. Journal of Clinical and Diagnostic Research. 2009;3(4):1653-1656.

[20] Fang H, Ataker F, Hedin G, Dornbusch K. Molecular epidemiology of extended-spectrum β-lactamases among *Escherichia coli* isolates in a Swedish hospital and its associated healthcare facilities in 2001-2006. Journal of Clinical Microbiology. 2007.

[21] Colodner R, Rock W, Chazan B, Keller N, Guy N, Sakran W, Raz R. Risk factors for the development of extended-spectrum beta-lactamase-producing bacteria in nonhospitalized patients. European Journal of Clinical Microbiology and Infectious Diseases. 2004;23(3):163-167.

[22] Magliano E, Grazioli V, Deflorio L, Leuci AI, Mattina R, Romano P, Cocuzza CE. Gender and age-dependent etiology of community-acquired urinary tract infections. The Scientific World Journal. 2012;2012.

[23] Calbo E, Romaní V, Xercavins M, Gómez L, Vidal CG, Quintana S, Vila J, Garau J. Risk factors for community-onset urinary tract infections due to *Escherichia coli* harbouring extended-spectrum β-lactamases. Journal of Antimicrobial Chemotherapy. 2006;57(4):780-783.

[24] Ena J, Arjona F, Martínez-Peinado C, del mar López-Perezagua M, Amador C. Epidemiology of urinary tract infections caused by extended-spectrum beta-lactamase-producing *Escherichia coli*. Urology. 2006;68(6):1169-1174.

[25] Cantas L, Suer K, Guler E, Imir T. High emergence of ESBL-producing *E. coli* cystitis: time to get smarter in Cyprus. Frontiers in Microbiology. 2016;6:1446.

[26] Mohamed ES, Khairy RM, Abdelrahim SS. Prevalence and molecular characteristics of ESBL and AmpC β-lactamase producing Enterobacteriaceae strains isolated from UTIs in Egypt. Antimicrobial Resistance & Infection Control. 2020;9(1):1-9.

[27] Yadav KK, Adhikari N, Khadka R, Pant AD, Shah B. Multidrug resistant Enterobacteriaceae and extended spectrum β-lactamase producing *Escherichia coli*: a cross-sectional study in National Kidney Center, Nepal. Antimicrobial Resistance and Infection Control. 2015;4(1):1-7.

[28] Chander A, Shrestha CD. Prevalence of extended spectrum beta lactamase

producing *Escherichia coli* and *Klebsiella pneumoniae* urinary isolates in a tertiary care hospital in Kathmandu, Nepal. BMC Research notes. 2013;6(1):1-6.

[29] Bhandari R, Pant ND, Poudel A, Sharma M. Assessment of the effectiveness of three different cephalosporin/clavulanate combinations for the phenotypic confirmation of extended-spectrum beta-lactamase producing bacteria isolated from urine samples at National Public Health Laboratory, Kathmandu, Nepal. BMC Research Notes. 2016;9(1):1-5.

Chapter 6

Post-Covid-19 Era: What is Next?

Shiela Chetri

Abstract

Antimicrobial resistance (AMR) is a natural phenomenon in bacteria which becomes a threat for health-care settings around the world. A concerted global response is needed to tackle rising rates of antibiotic resistance, without it we risk returning to the pre antibiotic era. As bacteria evolve very fast according to the environment in which they inhabit via developing different defence mechanisms to combat with the noxious agents like different classes of antibiotics including carbapenems. This results into treatment failure and clinical complications. Global emergence of antibiotic resistance due to bacterial multidrug efflux pump systems are a major and common mechanism of intrinsic antimicrobial resistance employed by bacteria which are spreading rapidly due to over use or misuse of antimicrobial agents. This review mainly focusses on the transcriptional expression of efflux pump system AcrAB-TolC, local regulatory genes (AcrR and AcrS), mediating carbapenem resistance in clinical isolates of *Escherichia coli* under antibiotic stress, a genetic interplay study between intrinsic and acquired antibiotic resistance mechanisms along with a brief summary on high risk factors and prevalence of urinary tract infections by multidrug resistant Uropathogenic *Escherichia coli*.

Keywords: *Escherichia coli*, carbapenem, AcrAB-TolC, $bla_{\text{NDM-1}}$, uropathogenic *Escherichia coli*

1. Introduction

Distribution of multi-drug resistant bacteria is a chief public health issue. Mutations have been an important factor influencing the development of the multi-drug resistant phenotypes and elucidate how they acquire antibiotic resistance [1, 2]. Several mutations are often required to acquire resistance towards a particular drug [3, 4]. However, a number of mechanisms evolved within bacteria helps them to survive against any noxious agents. Amongst the possible antibiotic resistance mechanisms, efflux pumps are membrane proteins which export noxious substances including antimicrobials out of the cell via over expressing the tripartite pump system resulting into antibiotic resistance [5]. Efflux pumps (like, AcrAB-TolC in *Escherichia coli* and MexAB-OprM in *P. aerugiosa*), are crucial for their survival and colonization/virulence, mainly during the development of infection when the pathogen is attacked by toxic substances or adhere with the host [6]. The AcrAB-TolC is constitutively expressed in *Escherichia coli*, and provides intrinsic resistance towards antimicrobials such as erythromycin and fusidic acid as well as dyes and detergents [7, 8]. In *Klebsiella pneumonia*, efflux pump mediated tigecycline resistance was reported from China in which higher expression of efflux pump systems AcrAB-TolC and OqxAB was recorded and the expression of AcrB gene was found to be connected with ramA and marA expression [9]. For decades, as a last resort carbapenems has been used quite effectively and the idea about this antibiotic was compromised due to the rise of carbapenem hydrolysing ß-Lactamase producers strain of *Klebsiella pneumoniae* [10]. Moreover, the situation is more convoluted in Indian subcontinent after appearance of New Delhi metallo-Beta lactamases in the present decade [11]. However, from India, in a study on *P. aeruginosa* isolates obtained from hospital revealed that MexAB-OprM efflux pump can considerably contribute to meropenem resistance in the absence of an acquired resistant mechanism [12]. According to a research done by Charleric B et al. 2003, clinical isolates of *Enterobacter aerogenes* exhibited resistance towards β-lactam and other group of antibiotics. Efflux pump associated resistance against quinolone, tetracycline and chloramphenicol along with over-expression of AcrA within these imipenem resistant strains have been observed earlier [13]. As per a study done by Chetri et al., 2019 a strong association between ertapenem resistance and AcrA over-expression was observed which has not been noticed earlier. Also, the over-expression of AcrB towards imipenem stress was noticed in this study is unique of its own [14]. AcrD, a transporter protein which belongs to RND superfamily of efflux pump was found to be associated with aminoglycosides resistance [15] did not show any role in carbapenem resistance in the above study [14]. Elkins and Nikaido in 2002, reported that for an efficient efflux of amphiphilic substrate, AcrD needs an association with AcrA in intact cells [16] and this association plays an important role in carbapenem non-susceptibility. Mutations in drug target genes are still presumed to be the crucial mechanism for drug resistance. To examine the basis of the increased expression of local regulators, AcrR and AcrS in AcrAB overexpressed isolates, mRNA sequencing of the regulatory regions was executed and was confirmed that the efflux pump mediated carbapenem resistance does not have any mutational event [16]. Dzwokai Ma and co-workers in 1996, reported that the transcriptional expression of AcrAB was increased under general stress condition and further, they investigated the role of the local repressor AcrR under general stress condition [16]. Remarkably, they found that under all these stress conditions, the transcription of AcrR was insistently increased and the level of increase was even higher than that observed for AcrA however, local repressor AcrR is associated as a repressor for AcrAB. In a study by Chetri and co-workers, the isolates with increased AcrAB expression under carbapenem stress showed much higher expression of AcrR which is surprising [14]. In agreement with the earlier study [14] it can be hypothesized that stress induced transcription of AcrAB is probably under the control of global transcriptional regulators.

New Delhi metallo beta-lactamase (NDM) is the predominant carbapenem resistance determinant in India which is harboured within members of enterobacteriaceae family and non-fermenters [17], and different variants have been reported from this country. Carbapenem resistance is a complex phenomenon which involves interplay between multiple acquired and intrinsic resistance mechanisms which includes loss or downregulation of porins, overexpression of different efflux pump systems and plasmid mediated acquirement of carbapenemase genes [18]. A previous study has noticed that efflux pump system plays an important role in carbapenem resistance compared to blaNDM-1 in *Pseudomonas aeruginosa* [18]. In another study, simultaneous expression of single component and multi component efflux pump was attempted in *E. coli* and *Pseudomonas aeruginosa* but it did not increase antibiotic resistance [19]. In similar work interplay between overexpression of AcrAB-TolC and mutation in gyrA and parC in quinolone resistance in *E. coli* was observed [20]. Also, a previous study has highlighted greater role of acrB in beta-lactam and quinolone resistance [21]. However, a study showed same pattern of transcriptional expression for both acrA and AcrB, which is probably due to the presence of both the genes in same transcript [22]. In a study done by Chetri et al., 2019 showed that in an *E. coli* isolate over-expressing both AcrAB-TolC and blaNDM-1, showed higher level of mRNA for both the genes when compared with other groups (II, III and IV) [22] and was observed that even a smaller amount of imipenem and meropenem was able to trigger the expression of NDM although; the role of ertapenem in induction was still unclear. Unlike *Pseudomonas aeruginosa*, where expression of efflux pump system MexAB-OprM was significant than that of blaNDM-1 [18], a study found contrasting pattern in *E. coli* [14]. In Indian subcontinent resistance against carbapenem is an evolving problem. However, acquirement of New Delhi metallo beta-lactamase is considered as the major reason for treatment failure and along with that efflux pump mediated resistance too remains a matter of concern as together both the mechanisms pose a grander risk. Study done by Chetri et al., 2019 was able to highlight a higher mRNA transcript of both the resistance genes when coexist within an isolate [22] and require further investigation to identify the concentration of antibiotics, duration of exposure and other factors responsible induction of these intrinsic and acquired mechanisms that exert an isolate a multidrug resistant phenotype.

Further, the active participation of *Escherichia coli* in causing Urinary tract infections, which is mainly caused by Uropathogenic *Escherichia coli* (UPEC) are the common bacterial infections [23]. In females, the high risk of UTIs is due to the intrinsic virulence of *E. coli* for colonization in urinary tract such as its capabilities to adhere to the tract and its association with other microorganisms moving from the perineum regions to the warmth moist environment of the female genitalia contaminated with fecal microbes [24, 25]. The worldwide rise of multi-drug resistant uropathogens, underscores the need for substitute non-antibiotic therapeutic and preventive approaches against Urinary tract infections.

However, a study done by Linsenmeyer et al. demonstrated a high level of indefinite empiric treatment for urinary tract infections caused by MDR gram-negative bacteria and patients suffering from MDR UTI is treated with an inactive antimicrobial agent as their preliminary therapy [26]. As in the previous study, estimation of non-fluoroquinolone antibiotics demonstrated the enhancement in accuracy of empiric therapy, considered as key concepts for stewardship programs [26]. Though, based upon the severity of illness, other patient factors and favoured means of drug administration, the therapeutic options can be selected. However, the high usage of fluoroquinolone is disturbing with the emergence of high resistance rates [27–29].

Other than *E. coli, Staphlylococcus aureus* which is a common cause of infections in health-care facilities and also in the community are part of our skin flora. A new AMR indicator was introduced in 2019 in the SDG monitoring framework which observes the frequency of bloodstream infections caused by two particular drug resistant microbes: *Escherichia coli* resistant to third generation cephalosporins and methicillin-resistant *Staphylococcus aureus (MRSA)*. Extensive resistance in extremely variable strains of *N. gonorrhoeae* has rapidly emerged and developed resistance towards macrolides, sulphonamides, fluoroquinolones, tetracyclines and early generation cephalosporins. The utilization of extended-spectrum cephalosporin ceftriaxone in injectable form are the only available therapeutic option for gonorrhoea in most countries currently. The threat of carbapenem resistant enterobacteriaceae (CRE) is emmerging and numerous mechanisms are associated in their non-susceptibility against carbapenem. This situation complicates the therapeutic scenario in critical care conditions in hospital setting as carbapenem resistant pathogens are most commonly found to be multidrug resistant. The epidemiology and occurrence rate of CRE differs in different geographical regions [30].

Antimicrobial resistance is an intricate issue which requires a combined multisectoral approach. One health approach brings together various divisions and stakeholders involved in human, aquatic and terrestrial animals and plants health, feed and food production and the environment to interact and work together for designing and execution of programmes and research to accomplish improved public health outcomes. The research and development of novel antimicrobials, vaccines and rapid diagnostic tools especially for targeting dangerous gram-negative bacteria like carbapenem resistant Enterobacteriaceae requires greater innovations and investments [30].

2. Conclusion

Multidrug efflux pumps are primeval elements encoded in the microorganism's chromosomes which confer resistance to antibiotics at different levels: intrinsic resistance, acquired resistance, and transient induced phenotypic resistance. Additionally, multidrug efflux pumps exhibit various functions with relevance to bacterial adaptation to altered habitats. Some of these functions, like resistance to heavy metals, resemble antibiotic resistance, biocides, or solvents, as they are adaptive responses to diverse types of external injuries, whereas, others are associated to internal detoxification of intermediate toxic bacterial metabolites. AcrAB pump is an important antibiotic resistance determinant in bacterial pathogen, having a dynamic role in developing resistance towards carbapenem group of antibiotics and the role of regulatory genes in inducing the expression of these pumps highlights the fact that the regulators directly or indirectly involved in increasing the expression of efflux pump system leading towards the development of carbapenem resistant MDR *Escherichia coli* isolates in clinical settings.

Acknowledgements

The authors would like to acknowledge Rajiv Gandhi South Campus, Banaras Hindu University for providing favourable environment and infrastructure facilities.

Conflict of interest

None.

Abbreviations

MDR	Multidrug Resistant
AMR	Antimicrobial resistance
CRE	carbapenem resistant Enterobacteriaceae
UTIs	Urinary tract infections
MRSA	methicillin-resistant *Staphylococcus aureus*
UPEC	Uropathogenic *Escherichia coli*
NDM	New Delhi metallo beta-lactamase

Author details

Shiela Chetri
Department of Microbiology, Faculty of Veterinary and Animal Sciences, Rajiv Gandhi South Campus, Banaras Hindu University, Barkachha, Mirzapur, Uttar Pradesh, India

*Address all correspondence to: sony240689@gmail.com

References

[1] Andersson DI, Hughes D. Antibiotic resistance and its cost: is it possible to reverse resistance?. Nature Reviews Microbiology. 2010 Apr;8(4):260-271.

[2] Toprak E, Veres A, Michel JB, Chait R, Hartl DL, Kishony R. Evolutionary paths to antibiotic resistance under dynamically sustained drug selection. Nature genetics. 2012 Jan;44(1):101-105.

[3] Weinreich DM, Delaney NF, DePristo MA, Hartl DL. Darwinian evolution can follow only very few mutational paths to fitter proteins. science. 2006 Apr 7;312(5770):111-114.

[4] Lozovsky ER, Chookajorn T, Brown KM, Imwong M, Shaw PJ, Kamchonwongpaisan S, Neafsey DE, Weinreich DM, Hartl DL. Stepwise acquisition of pyrimethamine resistance in the malaria parasite. Proceedings of the National Academy of Sciences. 2009 Jul 21;106(29):12025-12030.

[5] Piddock LJ. Multidrug-resistance efflux pumps? not just for resistance. Nature Reviews Microbiology. 2006 Aug;4(8):629-636.

[6] Zgurskaya HI, Nikaido H. Multidrug resistance mechanisms: drug efflux across two membranes. Molecular microbiology. 2000 Jul;37(2):219-225.

[7] Nikaido H. Multidrug efflux pumps of gram-negative bacteria. Journal of bacteriology. 1996 Oct;178(20):5853.

[8] Zhong X, Xu H, Chen D, Zhou H, Hu X, Cheng G. First emergence of acrAB and oqxAB mediated tigecycline resistance in clinical isolates of Klebsiella pneumoniae pre-dating the use of tigecycline in a Chinese hospital. PLoS One. 2014 Dec 12;9(12):e115185.

[9] Yigit H, Queenan AM, Rasheed JK, Biddle JW, Domenech-Sanchez A, Alberti S, Bush K, Tenover FC. Carbapenem-resistant strain of Klebsiella oxytoca harboring carbapenem-hydrolyzingβ-lactamase KPC-2. Antimicrobial agents and chemotherapy. 2003 Dec 1;47(12):3881-3889.

[10] Yong D, Toleman MA, Giske CG, Cho HS, Sundman K, Lee K, Walsh TR. Characterization of a new metallo-β-lactamase gene, blaNDM-1, and a novel erythromycin esterase gene carried on a unique genetic structure in Klebsiella pneumoniae sequence type 14 from India. Antimicrobial agents and chemotherapy. 2009 Dec 1;53(12):5046-5054.

[11] Choudhury D, Das Talukdar A, Dutta Choudhury M, Maurya AP, Paul D, Dhar Chanda D, Chakravorty A, Bhattacharjee A. Transcriptional analysis of MexAB-OprM efflux pumps system of Pseudomonas aeruginosa and its role in carbapenem resistance in a tertiary referral hospital in India. PLoS One. 2015 Jul 29;10(7):e0133842.

[12] Bornet C, Chollet R, Malléa M, Chevalier J, Davin-Regli A, Pagès JM, Bollet C. Imipenem and expression of multidrug efflux pump in Enterobacter aerogenes. Biochemical and biophysical research communications. 2003 Feb 21;301(4):985-990.

[13] Rosenberg EY, Ma D, Nikaido H. AcrD of Escherichia coli is an aminoglycoside efflux pump. Journal of bacteriology. 2000 Mar 15;182(6):1754-1756.

[14] Chetri S, Bhowmik D, Paul D, Pandey P, Chanda DD, Chakravarty A, Bora D, Bhattacharjee A. AcrAB-TolC efflux pump system plays a role in carbapenem non-susceptibility in Escherichia coli. BMC microbiology. 2019 Dec 1;19(1):210.

[15] Elkins CA, Nikaido H. Substrate specificity of the RND-type multidrug efflux pumps AcrB and AcrD of Escherichia coli is determined predominately by two large periplasmic loops. Journal of bacteriology. 2002 Dec 1;184(23):6490-6498.

[16] Ma D, Alberti M, Lynch C, Nikaido H, Hearst JE. The local repressor AcrR plays a modulating role in the regulation of acrAB genes of Escherichia coli by global stress signals. Molecular microbiology. 1996 Jan;19(1):101-112.

[17] Yong D, Toleman MA, Giske CG, Cho HS, Sundman K, Lee K, Walsh TR. Characterization of a new metallo-β-lactamase gene, blaNDM-1, and a novel erythromycin esterase gene carried on a unique genetic structure in Klebsiella pneumoniae sequence type 14 from India. Antimicrobial agents and chemotherapy. 2009 Dec 1;53(12):5046-5054.

[18] Choudhury D, Paul D, Ghosh AS, Talukdar AD, Choudhury MD, Maurya AP, Dhar D, Chakravarty A, Bhattacharjee A. Effect of single-dose carbapenem exposure on transcriptional expression of blaNDM-1 and mexA in Pseudomonas aeruginosa. Journal of Global Antimicrobial Resistance. 2016 Dec 1;7:72-77.

[19] Lee A, Mao W, Warren MS, Mistry A, Hoshino K, Okumura R, Ishida H, Lomovskaya O. Interplay between efflux pumps may provide either additive or multiplicative effects on drug resistance. Journal of bacteriology. 2000 Jun 1;182(11):3142-3150.

[20] Singh R, Swick MC, Ledesma KR, Yang Z, Hu M, Zechiedrich L, Tam VH. Temporal interplay between efflux pumps and target mutations in development of antibiotic resistance in Escherichia coli. Antimicrobial agents and chemotherapy. 2012 Apr 1;56(4):1680-1685.

[21] Padilla E, Llobet E, Doménech-Sánchez A, Martínez-Martínez L, Bengoechea JA, Albertí S. Klebsiella pneumoniae AcrAB efflux pump contributes to antimicrobial resistance and virulence. Antimicrobial agents and chemotherapy. 2010 Jan 1;54(1):177-183.

[22] Chetri S, Bhowmik D, Dhar D, Chakravarty A, Bhattacharjee A. Effect of concentration gradient carbapenem exposure on expression of blaNDM-1 and acrA in carbapenem resistant Escherichia coli. Infection, Genetics and Evolution. 2019 Sep 1;73:332-336.

[23] Loubet P, Ranfaing J, Dinh A, Dunyach-Remy C, Bernard L, Bruyère F, Lavigne JP, Sotto A. Alternative therapeutic options to antibiotics for the treatment of urinary tract infections. Frontiers in Microbiology. 2020;11.

[24] Andabati G, Byamugisha J. Microbial aetiology and sensitivity of asymptomatic bacteriuria among ante-natal mothers in Mulago hospital, Uganda. African health sciences. 2010;10(4).

[25] McLaughlin SP, Carson CC. Urinary tract infections in women. The Medical clinics of North America. 2004 Mar 1;88(2):417-429.

[26] Linsenmeyer K, Strymish J, Gupta K. Two simple rules for improving the accuracy of empiric treatment of multidrug-resistant urinary tract infections. Antimicrobial agents and chemotherapy. 2015 Dec 1;59(12):7593-7596.

[27] Ortega M, Marco F, Soriano A, Almela M, Martínez JA, Munoz A, Mensa J. Analysis of 4758 Escherichia coli bacteraemia episodes: predictive factors for isolation of an antibiotic-resistant strain and their

impact on the outcome. Journal of antimicrobial chemotherapy. 2009 Mar 1;63(3):568-574.

[28] MacVane SH, Tuttle LO, Nicolau DP. Impact of extended-spectrum β-lactamase–producing organisms on clinical and economic outcomes in patients with urinary tract infection. Journal of hospital medicine. 2014 Apr;9(4):232-238.

[29] MacFadden DR, Ridgway JP, Robicsek A, Elligsen M, Daneman N. Predictive utility of prior positive urine cultures. Clinical Infectious Diseases. 2014 Nov 1;59(9):1265-1271.

[30] https://www.who.int/news-room/fact-sheets/detail/antimicrobial-resistance

Chapter 7

Virulence and Antibiotic Resistance of *Acinetobacter baumannii* among Urinary Tract Infections

Hussein O.M. Al-Dahmoshi, Noor S.K. Al-Khafaji and Farah T. Al-Alaq

Abstract

Acinetobacter baumannii is one of the opportunistic bacteria firstly related with the hospital acquired infection influencing primarily to weakening the patient in the ICU. It is sometimes transferred to the patient by transient colonization of hands of the workers of healthcare, and persistence on eco-surfaces. Acinetobacter baumannii inhalation aerosolized through endo-tracheal suctioning of the ventilated patient is widespread among ventilator-related pneumonia (VAP). It is infections mainly associated with ventilator-related pneumonia (VAP), community Acquired Pneumonia (CAP), invasive bacterial infections (IBIs) and UTI (urinary tract infection). It is one of the prominent uropathogens problematic with antibiotic resistance especially carbapenem resistant Acinetobacter baumannii (CRAB). Their colonization of urinary tract and establishment of infection may attributed mainly to set of virulence factors like: Acinetobactin-assisted iron acquisition system, Bap (biofilm-related protein), phospholipase D, Ata (Acinetobacter trimeric autotransporter), chaperone-usher type pilus (Csu), OmpA (outer membrane protein A), and Plasminogen-binding protein (CipA). The common drugs used for treatment Acinetobacter baumannii infections involve polymyxins, glycylcyclines, tetracyclines, mono-bactams, fluoroquinolones, aminoglycosides, antipseudomonal carbapenems, antipseudomonal cephalosporins, and sulbactam. The rates of MDR isolation or also comprehensively the resistant Acinetobacter baumannii are significantly increased and so the combination of two or more (colistin, tigecycline, or colistin-rifampicin combination therapy) drugs is sometimes used to treat infections of MDR-AB. As a conclusion the Acinetobacter baumannii engagement in urinary tract infections attributed mainly to their adhesins, invasins and intrinsic antibiotic resistance.

Keywords: *A. baumannii*, CRAB, Ata, TAA, OmpA, CAP, VAP, colistin

1. Introduction

Acinetobacter baumannii is a polymorphic bacterium, rode shaped, gram negative, immobile, and aerobic. It is an opportunistic bacterium mainly related with the hospital acquired disease. It has highly incidence among immune-compromised people, especially those who have suffered from prolonged hospital stay (more than 90 days) [1]. A. baumannii bacterium is one of the major states of the infections of hospitals that firstly affect the exhausted patients in the ICU, notwithstanding the prevalence to long-term care facilities and to regular wards is becoming larger. It is distinguished by its great determination in environments and has a specially ability for enhancing the resistance to every antibiotic [2].

Acinetobacter baumannii usually causes the hospital infections, mostly catheter-related bacteremia, and aspiration pneumonia, but also can cause infections of urinary tract and soft tissue. Community-acquired infections Acinetobacter species are progressively recorded. Transfer of Acinetobacter, and sub-sequent diseases are expedited by environmental persistence of the microbes, resistance to dehydration and avoiding host immunity [3–5].

The characteristics of virulence exhibited by species of Acinetobacter mainly arises from avoiding of quick removal by the innate immunological system, actively expediting a highly bacterial density which leads to the formation of receptor of lipopolysaccharide-Toll-like 4 (TLR4)-assisted sepsis. Polysaccharides of capsule are critical virulence agents that enable immune evasion, whereas LPSs lead to the septic shock [6]. The newly increase in casualties, greatly related with the infected combat soldiers reverting from the conflict districts, and a high increasing in casualties of multidrug resistant isolates (MDRs) have increased the emerging opportunistic bacterium profile, significantly [7]. MDR-*A. baumannii*, defined as a strain resistant to 3 or more groups of antimicrobial agents. They are involving the carbapenem, which has emerged as a main cause of healthcare-related infection [8, 9]. The infections of A. baumannii are difficult for treating and related with highly, and mortality, and staying for a long time at hospitals [10, 11].

2. Acinetobacter spp.

Bacteria of the genus Acinetobacter are ubiquitous, free living, saprophytic organisms that can be isolated from soil, water, sewage, and a wide variety of foods. They are common components of food spoilage flora. *Acinetobacter johnsonii* and *Acinetobacter lwoffi* are the species most often isolated from foods, but other species, like the opportunistic pathogen *Acinetobacter baumannii* also can be found in spoilage flora [12]. *Acinetobacter* genus is very variant, consisting of negative and positive oxidase, non-pigmented, and gram negative cocco-bacilli. In spite of there are more than fifty species of the varied Acinetobacter, most of them are non-pathogenic environmental microorganisms. The most common infections are by A. baumannii, followed by A. lwoffii, and A. calcoaceticus [13, 14]. Acinetobacter was found out by Beigerinck, Martinus Willem, a microbiologist from Netherlands in 1911. However, for long times, the bacterium Acinetobacter had a low-virulence, sensitive to the used common antibiotics, but from 1970, resistance of Acinetobacter led to increase and became one of the severe problems, particularly in the conditions of hospitals. Currently, the infections by A. baumannii are distinguished to be an important problem and difficult for the controlling and treating in critical care conditions [15–17]. A. baumannii lives equally in the humid, and dry environments, is resistant to the disinfectant, and extreme drying. It enables for forming the biofilm that expedites bacterial binding to the tissue, as well as different surfaces of the environment, and rapidly acquires mechanisms of the antibiotic resistance. These characteristics are believed to have led to the quick endemic prevalence of Acinetobacter baumannii in environments of hospitals and several intensive care units worldwide, especially in countries of Europe. Also, in 2015, the report of the European Antimicrobial Resistance Control Network referred to that the association of strains of MRD-A. baumannii throughout Europe was stably increasing.

However, the highest levels of the drug resistance Acinetobacter baumannii were remarked in the states of Baltic particularly in Lithuania and in Southeastern and Southern Europe. In 2017, this bacterial species was involved in the general priority list of WHO for drug-resistant bacteria for a big need to the development of research, and the insistence for novel antimicrobial agents [18]. *Acinetobacter* spp. are normally dwell skin, mucous membranes or the pharynx, and human respiratory secretions as normal flora It accountable for a wide variety of local and systemic infections, including pneumonia, septicemia, wound infections and urinary tract infections. The main body areas populated by these microorganisms in hospitalized patients are the skin, oropharynx, and digestive tract [19–21]. Additionally it can survive in dry abiotic environment like medical devices, disposables mattresses, pillows and equipment for long periods. It can stay on glass for 20 days and their staying on another dry surface may be 4 moths [22].

3. Urinary tract infections

A. baumannii infections involve body systems that with high levels of fluids such as urinary and respiratory tract, peritoneal cavity, and are linked to indwelling devices [21]. The UTI (Urinary tract infection) has a main public health concern in sciences of medicine and represents one of the most commonly infectious diseases classified next to infections of the upper respiratory tract. They precipitate to nosocomial infections in several hospitals and account approx. 35% of all diseases obtained in the hospitals. Unhealthy lacks of proper genital washing and sexual intercourse have led to spread UTI. [23]. Genitourinary infections regards third important hospital infections proceed by respiratory and surgical wound infections A. baumannii responsible for 5-9% of UTIS [24–26].

A. baumannii compile 1-2% of all healthcare-related infections in the USA, Europe and Middle East [27]. A. baumannii Catheter associated UTIs (CAUTI) is most recently UTIs rerated to biofilm formation among uropathogens. A. baumannii was implicated as uropathogens and 20% of all isolates were isolated from patients with UTIs [28]. This organism is usually linked to catheter-associated infection or colonization. It is unusual for *A. baumannii* to cause complicated UTI in outpatients. Epidemiologically MDR-AB were widespread worldwide: Europe, North America, Argentina, Brazil, China, Taiwan, Hong Kong, Japan, and Korea [29–31]. Cross-transmission and diffusion from the hospital environment are more likely than endogenous sources to be the source of infecting or colonizing organisms in nosocomial infections [32]. *A. baumannii* very dangerous specially in individuals who have recently undergone major surgery, have malignant diseases or burns or immuno-suppressed patients such as the elderly, neonates with low birth weights, and patients with prolonged illnesses [33]. War-associated infections was clearly linked to *A. baumannii* when reported during the Korean War, the Vietnam War, and the wars in Iraq and Afghanistan [34, 35]. Biofilm formation were investigated among more than 75% of A. baumannii isolates and it can bind to the host epithelial cells via set of adhesins like Csu, OmpA and Bap [36–39].

4. Virulence factors

The interaction between cells of the host and pathogens is important in the pathogenesis of some bacteria leads to its internalization. Although proving the infections, the bacteria must be colonizing the host. The binding of pathogens to cells of the host is enhanced by different molecules expression or structures by cells of bacteria. Adhesion depends on the interferences of proteins of the host cell surface or soluble proteins with receptors. The proteins act as a bridge between cells of the host and bacteria. Adherence of microbes to cells of the host as a first step of colonization is an important virulence agent [40, 41]. Few molecular agents are needed to the virulence of A. baumannii in human. They involve excessively phospholipase D, OmpA (outer membrane protein A), Csu (chaperone usher type pilus), Bap (biofilm associated protein), acinetobactin assisted Fe acquisition system, and Ata (Acinetobacter trimeric autotransporter), [42]. The role of each of them in virulence was listed below:

4.1 Bap (biofilm-associated protein)

In vitro, cells of A. baumannii easily form the biofilm, and the capability of nosocomial strains for forming the biofilm on the medical devices as in tissues of the host finds a critical agent in the virulence of bacteria. The cells that synthesize the biofilms are included in the polymeric conglomerate of polysaccharides and proteins. The biofilm resists immune defenses of the host, antibiotics and detergents, and antibiotic resistance to bacteria in these habitats can be increased to 1000 times [43, 44]. The biofilm finally grows by producing poly-beta (1-6) N-acetyl-glucosamine controlled by pgalocus. The extracellular matrix gives an adhesion among the cells of bacteria, allowing the synthesis of multilayer structures. Also, many surface proteins are included in the process, and show to expressively contribute to the binding of the bacterial cells to abiotic or biological surfaces. Directly, Bap (biofilm associated protein), a special cell surface protein, is included in the formation of the biofilm by Acinetobacter baumannii and plays a main role in the processes of infectious bacteria. It is involved in intercellular adhesion within the mature biofilm [45]. Bap (Acinetobacter baumannii biofilm-related protein) is necessary to form a mature biofilm on the medically-relevant surfaces, involving polystyrene, titanium, and polypropylene, and Bap acts as the surface structure included in A. baumannii adherence to normal human neonatal keratinocytes and normal human bronchial epithelial cells. The finding Bap increases hydrophobicity of surface of the cell of bacteria [46]. Bap is A giant protein plays a great role in the formation of biofilms and adhesion to cells of the host in A. baumannii. Most of the protein is synthesized by arrays of 80 to 110 modules featuring Ig-like (immunoglobulin-like) motifs. Bap types includes BLP1, and BLP2 which included in the formation of biofilms and assembled in dissimilar A. baumannii isolates. However, adhesion patterns and phenotypes of the biofilm of some clinical strains appear to be associated with the finding broadspectrum antibiotic resistances. Also, the arrangement of the development, and formation of the biofilms diverse like surfaces on which these bacteria persist and components of cells that contribute in the multi-step programmed process. The regulatory processes related with the synthesis of biofilms involve sensing density of the cells of bacteria, the finding various nutrients and concentrations of free cations found for the cells of bacteria. Extracellularly, some of the signals maybe sensed by 2 component regulatory systems like Bfm RS. The transcriptional regulatory system activates expressions of usher-chaperone assembly systems accountable to produce pili, needed for the synthesis of the biofilms on the polystyrene surfaces, and cell attachment. Nevertheless, this system is not required for the formation of biofilms on abiotic surfaces when the cells are cultured in the industrial medium. Interestingly, system of Bfm RS controls the shape of the cell under certain cultural setting. Biofilm tolerance to host immune defenses, disinfectants, and antimicrobials [47, 48].

4.2 OmpA (Outer membrane protein A)

The main protein of outer membranes, (OmpA), is the most abundant surface protein. Also, it is necessary to bind A. baumannii to human alveolar epithelium, but it also plays a useful role in the enhancement of biofilms on plastics. Among the identified proteins of outer membrane in A. baumannii, AbOmpA acts as a porin, which is required for adhesion of eukaryotic cells, and participates to resistance of serum and the biofilm formation, partially. The OmpA group is proposed to have a variety of functions, involving adhesion to epithelial cells of the host, functions of biofilms, and complement resistance [49]. Additionally, overexpression of chromosomal efflux systems was received great attention. However, the over-production of these systems confers increased MDR to antibacterial factors and induces death of cells of the host through nuclear and mitochondrial targeting [50–52]. OmpA thought to participate to the antibacteral resistance of *A. baumannii* during a probable interaction between efflux pump systems and its OmpA-like domain [53].

4.3 Phospholipase D

PL (Phospholipase) is an essential enzyme, necessary for phosphatidylcholine metabolism and was studied in a variety spectrum of microbes. About, 3 phospholipase classes (PLC, PLD, and PLA) were identified by the cleavage site. PLA analyzes the fatty acid of the glycerol backbone. When PLC cleavage, the phosphorylated head groups are released from PLD and phospholipid cleaves off just the head group. The releasing the polar head group and the releasing the phosphorylated head group can affect the constancy of membranes of the host cells. Additionally, phospholipase can interfere with cellular signaling by generating 2nd messengers such as phosphatidic acid, which can modify the immune responses of the host [54]. It is assumed that many pathogens exploit certain enzymes for enhancement of membranes in the coordinated form, thus, these enzymes play an important role as virulent agents. An example is PLD (phospholipase D), an enzyme that hydrolyses structural phospholipids which results in PA (phosphatidic acid) production, a 2nd messenger that acts as an assistor in several cellular processes. Phospholipase as a virulence agent was implicated in many bacteria. In vivo, PLD of A. baumannii supports pathogenesis and invasion [55, 56]. The disrupting A. baumannii phospholipase D caused reducing capability of organisms to grow in the blood serum, decreased pathogenesis and decreasing epithelial cell invasion [57].

4.4 Csu (chaperone-usher type pilus)

The attachment of primary cell can be reasonably assisted by a pili -like structure encoded by the position of csu, which is widely spread among clinical strains. A. baumannii ability to form the biofilm largely depends on pilus, which assists formation and attachment of biofilms. In similar, csu E, is one of the members of the system of usher-chaperone. Genes clustered together in the form of opera csu, whose products form pili-like bundle structures in these bacteria. This gene has confirmed to be a meaningful agent in the formation of A. baumannii biofilm [58, 59].

4.5 Acinetobacter trimeric autotransporter (Ata)

The Ata (Acinetobacter Trimeric automatic transmission adhesive) pertains to the trimeric autotransporter adhesin super-family which is meaningful virulence agents in several gram negative pathogens. Also, the TAA (Trimeric autotransporter), called as the Vc type secretion system, is declared by several A. baumannii isolates, an opportunistic bacteria, answerable for the infections in hospitals globally. The TAA, is a modular homotrimeric virulence agent, including conserved membrane anchoring domain, the signal peptide, and complex stalk. In vivo, mechanisms of the evolutionary underlying the development of this adhesin is not clear. The Ata is an useful multi-functional virulence agent in the bacterium Acinetobacter baumannii that assists the invasion and the adhesion, participates with pathogenicity, and incites apoptosis [60]. It was found that the Ata is acting as a multi-functional virulence agent of Acinetobacter baumannii by (1) mediating the invasion and adhesion in cells of epithelial and endothelial, (2) leading to the programmed cell death in a caspas-dependent manner, (3) leading to the secreting IL-6 and IL-8 as proinflammatory cytokines, and (4) in vivo, contributes to the virulence. These results forcefully propose that The Ata was uses as useful virulence factors for the bacterium Acinetobacter baumannii through the infections in models of insect and human [61].

4.6 System of Acinetobactin-assisted iron acquisition

The siderophore is highly converged iron chelators synthesized and applied using some bacteria to thrive under the iron-reducing which conditions typically encountered in hosts and the environment [62]. A. baumannii produces up to 3 siderophores namely, baumannoferrin, fimsbactin, and acinetobactin. The producing baumannoferrin, and acinetobactin is beggarly conserved among clinical strains, whereas the producting fimsbactin is lesser common. Fimsbactins are structurally linked to acinetobactin by the finding catecholate, and phenolate oxazoline metal binding motifs. Both are derived from nonribosomal peptide synthesis lines with similar catalytic domain, identities, and orientations [63]. The system of acetinopactin-assisted iron acquisition was the most distinctive system in Acinetobacter baumannii. Acinetobactins, catechol-hydroxamate siderophores, and non cyclic derivative of DHBA, that associated with N-hydroxyhistamine, and threonine. Acinetobactins are synthesized and used by 3 hypothetical systems encoded within the gene clusters of acinetobactin in Acinetobacter baumannii. Acinetobactins are manufactured from threonine, hydroxy histamine, and DHBA by the encoded proteins by genes in the gene cluster. The mixed kind siderophore, which constitutes of hydroxamite groups and catechols groups, shows a significant affinity of Fe. Acinetobacter baumannii that is produced acinetobactin is secreted system of the siderophore efflux the super-family of ABC [64].

4.7 CipA (plasminogen binding protein)

The CipA (Plasminogen-binding protein) is an external membrane protein, links to active forms of the plasmin, and plasminogen, to break down fibrinogen and encourage the spread of bacteria. Also, this CipA plasmin breaks down C3b. Nevertheless, there is no correlation among CipA plasmin levels, and complement resistance so far. Thus, the mechanism by which CipA gives the complement resistance still needs clarification. The CipA disrupts the system of alternative supplements and supports the penetration of layers of endothelium [65].

5. Antibiotic resistance and therapeutics options

A. baumannii remains difficult for treatment that has an important challenge to the clinician and cost to the systems of healthcare. Commonly, the used antibiotics to treat infections of Acinetobacter baumannii involve polymyxins, glycylcyclines, tetracyclines, fluoroquinolones, aminoglycosides, mono-bactams, antipseudomonal carbapenems, antipseudomonal cephalosporins, and sulbactam [66]. Colistin was widely investigated as a mono-therapy or as a part of the combination treatment, but its application is limited because of the nephrotoxicity. Previously, infections of Acinetobacter baumannii to CNS (central nervous system) following neurosurgery were recorded and treated with relative success by tigecycline, colistin, intraventricular or/and intravenous or colistin-rifampicin combination thretment [67]. Application of Colistin exhibits an upward tendency because of the VAP overseas and emergence of the bacterial infections of MDR [68]. Nevertheless, none of tigecycline or polymyxins was excessively agreed for the medical uses in China. Actually, using combinations of beta-lactamase inhibitor (sulbactam/ampicillin and sulbactam/cefoperazone) or meropenem as the basis of the therapy program associated by levofloxacin or etilmicin is repeatedly used in therapies of the empiric antibiotics. Recently, broad spectrum antibiotics were greatly applied in the clinical practices, whereas the rate Acinetobacter baumannii resistance shows obvious increases [69, 70]. Significantly, the rates resistant Acinetobacter baumannii of or even comprehensively MDR isolation are increased in clinic. The studies were exhibited that the rate resistance of Acinetobacter baumannii to most the tested antibiotics is more than 50%. Thus, the combination of two or more antibiotics is sometimes used in treatment of the infections of MDR-AB [71, 72].

However, due to its widespread use, resistance of AB to carbapenem antibiotics quickly increased, in particular among isolates obtained from the ICU. In China, the incidence of resistance of carbapenem (CRAB) increased from the percentage 31% in 2005 to the percentage 66.7% in 2014. In USA, it increased from the percentage 20.6% in 2002 to the percentage 49.2% in 2008. Very few drugs are now available to treat CRAB (carbapenem resistant AB). It is hypersensitive to just a few drugs, like tigecycline and polymyxin, in vitro [73–75].

Currently, the best therapy for the infections of CRAB is illegible. In China, tigecycline based combination treatment, polymyxin based combination treatment, and sulbactam based combination treatment are devised to treat MDR Gram negative rode bacteria. Nevertheless, these devises are based on small scale retrospective researches, lacking comprehensive and systematic clinical study evidence, and no large scale clinical randomized controlled trials were achieved to assess their activity in the patient with MDR-A. baumannii. Polymyxin is not greatly applied in Mainland China because of the toxic side influences of it [76, 77]. Thus, currently, tigecycline treatment and sulbactam treatment are the major clinical therapies for CRAB. Nevertheless, several controversies surround tigecycline regimen to treat infections of A. baumannii bloodstream (BSI). The US Food and Drug Administration devised that tigecycline was autonomously related with highly risks of mortality and must just be applied in conditions where therapeutic preferences were limited. However, tigecycline exerts a suitable therapeutic influence depending to some researches, whereas many other researches recorded that tigecycline increases the mortality of patient [78, 79].

As a member of Gram negative bacteria, A. baumannii equipped with sets of resistance mechanisms including: i) structural bacterial shields (Presence of the porin channels and efflux mechanisms), ii) enzymatic inactivation of antibiotics (oxacillinase (OXA-type), metallo–beta-lactamases (MBLs), iii) alteration of the target or cellular functions due to mutations [80–82].

Due to extensive resistance to antibiotics, new strategies were proposed as alternative therapy. Antimicrobial peptides (AMPs) are one of the antimicrobial agents with high potential to produce new anti-*Acinetobacter* drugs. Melittin, Histatin-8,

Omega76, AM-CATH36, Hymenochirin, and Mastoparan were suitaple AMPs and have the highest anti-*A. baumannii* [83–85].

Pahge or bacteriophage therapy is another alternative therapy for MDRAP. Phages are specific to different bacteria, and they bind to receptors on bacterial cell walls to inject deoxyribonucleic acid into the cell and ultimately lyse the cell in the lytic phase. Lytic bacteriophage therapy may be an opportunity to combat the rapidly growing number of MDR bacteria [86]. Lytic phage, the YMC 13/03/R2096 ABA BP (phage BΦ-R2096), which specifically causes the lysis of CRAB strains [87].

6. Conclusion

As a conclusion the Acinetobacter baumannii engagement in urinary tract infections attributed mainly to their adhesins, invasins and intrinsic antibiotic resistance.

Conflict of interest

There is no 'conflict of interest' for this work.

Author details

Hussein O.M. Al-Dahmoshi*, Noor S.K. Al-Khafaji and Farah T. Al-Alaq
Department of Biology, College of Science, University of Babylon, Hilla, Iraq

*Address all correspondence to: dr.dahmoshi83@gmail.com

References

[1] Montefour, K., Frieden, J., Hurst, S., Helmich, C., Headley, D., Martin, M. and Boyle, D.A., 2008. Acinetobacter baumannii: an emerging multidrug-resistant pathogen in critical care. Critical care nurse, 28(1), pp. 15-25.

[2] Garnacho-Montero, J. and Timsit, J.F., 2019. Managing Acinetobacter baumannii infections. Current opinion in infectious diseases, 32(1), pp. 69-76.

[3] Dexter, C., Murray, G.L., Paulsen, I.T. and Peleg, A.Y., 2015. Community-acquired Acinetobacter baumannii: clinical characteristics, epidemiology and pathogenesis. Expert review of anti-infective therapy, 13(5), pp. 567-573.

[4] Zilberberg, M.D., Nathanson, B.H., Sulham, K., Fan, W. and Shorr, A.F., 2016. Multidrug resistance, inappropriate empiric therapy, and hospital mortality in Acinetobacter baumannii pneumonia and sepsis. Critical Care, 20(1), p.221.

[5] Liu, A., Du, W., Xie, J., Qiu, H. and Yang, Y., 2018. 720: Deficiency Of Cdc In Immunocompromised Mice With Acinetobacter Baumannii Pneumonia. Critical Care Medicine, 46(1), p.346.

[6] Wong, D., Nielsen, T.B., Bonomo, R.A., Pantapalangkoor, P., Luna, B. and Spellberg, B., 2017. Clinical and pathophysiological overview of Acinetobacter infections: a century of challenges. Clinical microbiology reviews, 30(1), pp.409-447.

[7] Howard, A., O'Donoghue, M., Feeney, A. and Sleator, R.D., 2012. Acinetobacter baumannii: an emerging opportunistic pathogen. Virulence, 3(3), pp.243-250.

[8] Munoz-Price, L.S. and Weinstein, R.A., 2008. Acinetobacter infection. New England Journal of Medicine, 358(12), pp.1271-1281.

[9] Peleg, A.Y., Seifert, H. and Paterson, D.L., 2008. Acinetobacter baumannii: emergence of a successful pathogen. Clinical microbiology reviews, 21(3), pp.538-582.

[10] Magill, S.S., Edwards, J.R., Bamberg, W., Beldavs, Z.G., Dumyati, G., Kainer, M.A., Lynfield, R., Maloney, M., McAllister-Hollod, L., Nadle, J. and Ray, S.M., 2014. Multistate point-prevalence survey of health care–associated infections. New England Journal of Medicine, 370(13), pp.1198-1208.

[11] Ainsworth, S., Ketter, P.M., Yu, J.J., Grimm, R.C., May, H.C., Cap, A.P., Chambers, J.P., Guentzel, M.N. and Arulanandam, B.P., 2017. Vaccination with a live attenuated Acinetobacter baumannii deficient in thioredoxin provides protection against systemic Acinetobacter infection. Vaccine, 35(26), pp.3387-3394.

[12] Robinson RK. Encyclopedia of food microbiology. Academic press; 2014 Apr 2.

[13] Al Atrouni A, Joly-Guillou ML, Hamze M, Kempf M. 2016. Reservoirs of non-baumannii Acinetobacter species. Front Microbiol 7:49.

[14] Mohanty, A., Kabi, A. and Mohanty, A.P., 2018. Acinetobacterlwoffii-Emerging pathogen causing liver abscess: A Case Report. National Journal of Integrated Research in Medicine, 9(5), pp.53-54.

[15] Niederman, M.S.; Kollef, M.H. The road forward in the management of Acinetobacter infections in ICU. Intensive Care Med. 2015, 41, 2207-2209.

[16] Garnacho-Montero, J.; Gutierrez-Pizarraya, A.; Diaz-Martin, A.; Cisneros-Herreros, J.M.; Cano,

M.E.; Gato, E.; Ruiz de Alegría, C.; Fernández-Cuenca, F.; Vila, J.; Martínez-Martínez, L.; et al. Acinetobacter baumannii in critically ill patients: Molecular epidemiology, clinical features and predictors of mortality. Enferm. Infecc. Microbiol. Clin. 2016, 34, 551-558.

[17] Rello, J.; Kalwaje Eshwara, K.; Lagunes, L.; Alves, J.; Wunderic, R.G.; Conway-Morris, A.; Rojas, J.N.; Alp, E.; Zhang, Z. A global priority list of the TOp TEn resistant Microorganisms (TOTEM) study at intensive care: A prioritization exercise based on multi-criteria decision analysis. Eur. J. Clin. Microbiol. Infect. Dis. 2019, 38, 319-323.

[18] European Centre for Disease Prevention and Control. European Antibiotic Awareness Day (EAAD) Summary of the Latest Data on Antibiotic Resistance in the European Union; EARS-Net Surveillance Data 2015; ECDC: Stockholm, Sweden, 2016.

[19] Towner K. The genus acinetobacter. Prok. 2006;6:746-58.

[20] Munoz-Price LS, Weinstein RA. Acinetobacter infection. New England Journal of Medicine. 2008 Mar 20;358(12):1271-81.

[21] Jung J, Park W. Acinetobacter species as model microorganisms in environmental microbiology: current state and perspectives. Applied microbiology and biotechnology. 2015 Mar 1;99(6):2533-48.

[22] Lee K, Yong D, Jeong SH, Chong Y. Multidrug-resistant Acinetobacter spp.: increasingly problematic nosocomial pathogens. Yonsei medical journal. 2011 Nov 1;52(6):879-91.

[23] Flores-Mireles A.L., J. .N. Walker, M. Caparon, S.J. Hultgren, Urinary tract infections: epidemiology, mechanisms of infection and treatment options, Nature Rev. Microbiol. 13 (2015) 269-284.

[24] Patel, H.B., Soni, S.T., Bhagyalaxmi, A. and Patel, N.M., 2019. Causative agents of urinary tract infections and their antimicrobial susceptibility patterns at a referral center in Western India: An audit to help clinicians prevent antibiotic misuse. Journal of Family Medicine and Primary Care, 8(1), p.154.

[25] Baviskar, A.S., Khatib, K.I., Rajpal, D. and Dongare, H.C., 2019. Nosocomial infections in surgical intensive care unit: A retrospective single-center study. International Journal of Critical Illness and Injury Science, 9(1), p.16.

[26] Presterl, E., Diab-El Schahawi, M., Lusignani, L.S., Paula, H. and Reilly, J.S., 2019. Hospital Infections. In Basic Microbiology and Infection Control for Midwives (pp. 85-91). Springer, Cham.

[27] Lob SH, Hoban DJ, Sahm DF, Badal RE. Regional differences and trends in antimicrobial susceptibility of Acinetobacter baumannii. International journal of antimicrobial agents. 2016 Apr 1;47(4):317-23. Stickler DJ. Bacterial biofilms in patients with indwelling urinary catheters. Nature clinical practice urology. 2008 Nov;5(11):598-608.

[28] Di Venanzio G, Flores-Mireles AL, Calix JJ, Haurat MF, Scott NE, Palmer LD, Potter RF, Hibbing ME, Friedman L, Wang B, Dantas G. Urinary tract colonization is enhanced by a plasmid that regulates uropathogenic Acinetobacter baumannii chromosomal genes. Nature communications. 2019 Jun 24;10(1):1-3.

[29] Lolans K, Rice TW, Munoz-Price LS, Quinn JP. Multicity outbreak of carbapenem-resistant Acinetobacter baumannii isolates producing the carbapenemase OXA-40. Antimicrobial agents and chemotherapy. 2006 Sep 1;50(9):2941-5.

[30] Coelho JM, Turton JF, Kaufmann ME, Glover J, Woodford N, Warner M, Palepou MF, Pike R, Pitt TL, Patel BC, Livermore DM. Occurrence of carbapenem-resistant Acinetobacter baumannii clones at multiple hospitals in London and Southeast England. Journal of clinical microbiology. 2006 Oct 1;44(10):3623-7.

[31] Siempos II, Vardakas KZ, Kyriakopoulos CE, Ntaidou TK, Falagas ME. Predictors of mortality in adult patients with ventilator-associated pneumonia: a meta-analysis. Shock. 2010 Jun 1;33(6):590-601.

[32] Luna CM, Aruj PK. Nosocomial acinetobacter pneumonia. Respirology. 2007 Nov;12(6):787-91.

[33] Doughari HJ, Ndakidemi PA, Human IS, Benade S. The ecology, biology and pathogenesis of Acinetobacter spp.: an overview. Microbes and environments. 2009:1103150282-.

[34] Scott P, Deye G, Srinivasan A, Murray C, Moran K, Hulten E, Fishbain J, Craft D, Riddell S, Lindler L, Mancuso J. An outbreak of multidrug-resistant Acinetobacter baumannii-calcoaceticus complex infection in the US military health care system associated with military operations in Iraq. Clinical Infectious Diseases. 2007 Jun 15;44(12):1577-84.

[35] Sheppard FR, Keiser P, Craft DW, Gage F, Robson M, Brown TS, Petersen K, Sincock S, Kasper M, Hawksworth J, Tadaki D. The majority of US combat casualty soft-tissue wounds are not infected or colonized upon arrival or during treatment at a continental US military medical facility. The American journal of surgery. 2010 Oct 1;200(4):489-95.

[36] AziziO,ShahcheraghiF,SalimizandH, Modarresi F, Shakibaie MR, Mansouri S, Ramazanzadeh R, Badmasti F, Nikbin V. Molecular analysis and expression of bap gene in biofilm-forming multi-drug-resistant Acinetobacter baumannii. Reports of biochemistry & molecular biology. 2016 Oct;5(1):62.

[37] Greene C, Wu J, Rickard AH, Xi C. Evaluation of the ability of Acinetobacter baumannii to form biofilms on six different biomedical relevant surfaces. Letters in applied microbiology. 2016 Oct;63(4):233-9.

[38] Zeighami H, Valadkhani F, Shapouri R, Samadi E, Haghi F. Virulence characteristics of multidrug resistant biofilm forming Acinetobacter baumannii isolated from intensive care unit patients. BMC infectious diseases. 2019 Dec;19(1):629.

[39] Falagas ME, Vardakas KZ, Kapaskelis A, Triarides NA, Roussos NS. Tetracyclines for multidrug-resistant Acinetobacter baumannii infections. International journal of antimicrobial agents. 2015 May 1;45(5):455-60.

[40] Smani Y, McConnell MJ, Pachon J. Role of fibronectin in the adhesion of Acinetobacter baumannii to host cells. PLoS One. 2012;7(4). e33073.

[41] Vijayakumar S, Rajenderan S, Laishram S, Anandan S, Balaji V, Biswas I. Biofilm Formation and Motility Depend on the Nature of the Acinetobacter baumannii Clinical Isolates. Front Public Health. 2016;4:105.

[42] Harding CM, Tracy EN, Carruthers MD, Rather PN, Actis LA, Munson RS Jr. Acinetobacter baumannii strain M2 produces type IV pili which play a role in natural transformation and twitching motility but not surface-associated motility. MBio. 2013;4(4).

[43] Giannouli M, Antunes LCS, Marchetti V, Triassi M, Visca P, Zarrilli R. Virulence-related traits of epidemic Acinetobacter baumannii

strains belonging to the international clonal lineages I-III and to the emerging genotypes ST25 and ST78. BMC Infect Dis. 2013;13:282.

[44] Longo F, Vuotto C, Donelli G. Biofilm formation in Acinetobacter baumannii. New Microbiol. 2014;37:119-27.

[45] Fattahian, Y., Rasooli, I., Gargari, S.L.M., Rahbar, M.R., Astaneh, S.D.A. and Amani, J., 2011. Protection against Acinetobacter baumannii infection via its functional deprivation of biofilm associated protein (Bap). Microbial pathogenesis, 51(6), pp.402-406.

[46] Brossard, K.A. and Campagnari, A.A., 2012. The Acinetobacter baumannii biofilm-associated protein plays a role in adherence to human epithelial cells. Infection and immunity, 80(1), pp.228-233.

[47] Gaddy, Jennifer A., and Luis A. Actis. "Regulation of Acinetobacter baumannii biofilm formation." (2009): 273-278.

[48] Sefid, F., Rasooli, I. and Payandeh, Z., 2016. Homology modeling of a Camelid antibody fragment against a conserved region of Acinetobacter baumannii biofilm associated protein (Bap). Journal of theoretical biology, 397, pp.43-51.

[49] Schweppe DK, Harding C, Chavez JD, Wu X, Ramage E, Singh PK, Manoil C, Bruce JE. 2015. Host-microbe protein interactions during bacterial infection. Chem Biol 22:1521-1530.

[50] Richmond GE, Evans LP, Anderson MJ, Wand ME, Bonney LC, IvensA, ChuaKL, WebberMA, SuttonJM, Peterson ML, Piddock LJ. 2016. The Acinetobacterbaumanniitwo-component system AdeRS regulates genes required for multidrug efflux, biofilm formation, and virulence in a strain-specific manner. mBio 7:e00430-16.

[51] Yoon EJ, Balloy V, Fiette L, Chignard M, Courvalin P, Grillot-Courvalin C. 2016. Contribution of the Ade resistance-nodulation-cell division-type efflux pumps to fitness and pathogenesis of Acinetobacter baumannii. mBio 7:e00697-16.

[52] Ismail, L.I.M., 2019. Studies on OmpA of Acinetobacter baumannii in Virulence and Immunity in a Cell Culture Model. CU Theses.

[53] Kwon H. I., S. Kim, M.H. Oh, S.H. Na, Y.J.Kim, Y.H. Jeon, J.C. LeeOuter membrane protein A contributes to antimicrobial resistance of Acinetobacter baumannii through the OmpA-like domain J. Antimicrob. Chemother., 72 (2017), pp. 3012-3015.

[54] Selvy PE, Lavieri RR, Lindsley CW, Brown HA. Phospholipase D: enzymology, functionality, and chemical modulation. Chem Rev. 2011;111: 6064-6119

[55] Köhler, G.A., Brenot, A., Haas-Stapleton, E., Agabian, N., Deva, R. and Nigam, S. (2006)Phospholipase A(2) and phospholipase B activities in fungi. Biochim. Biophys. Acta, 1761, 1391– 1399.

[56] Stahl J, Bergmann H, Göttig S, et al. Acinetobacter baumannii virulence is mediated by the concerted action of three phospholipases D. PLoS ONE. 2015;10:e0138360.

[57] Jacobs, A.C., Hood, I., Boyd, K.L., Olson, P.D., Morrison, J.M., Carson, S., Sayood, K., Iwen, P.C., Skaar, E.P. and Dunman, P.M., 2010. Inactivation of phospholipase D diminishes Acinetobacter baumannii pathogenesis. Infection and immunity, 78(5), pp.1952-1962.

[58] Lee HW, Koh Y, Kim J, Lee JC, Lee YC, Seol SY, et al. Capacity of multidrug-resistant clinical isolates of Acinetobacter baumannii to form

biofilm and adhere to epithelial cell surfaces. Clin Microbiol Infec. 2008;14:49-54.

[59] Tomaras AP, Flagler MJ, Dorsey CW, Gaddy JA, Actis LA. Characterization of a two-component regulatory system from Acinetobacter baumannii that controls biofilm formation and cellular morphology. Microbiology. 2008;154:3398-409.

[60] Rahbar, M.R., Zarei, M., Jahangiri, A., Khalili, S., Nezafat, N., Negahdaripour, M., Fattahian, Y. and Ghasemi, Y., 2019. Trimeric autotransporter adhesins in Acinetobacter baumannii, coincidental evolution at work. Infection, Genetics and Evolution.

[61] Weidensdorfer, M., Ishikawa, M., Hori, K., Linke, D., Djahanschiri, B., Iruegas, R., Ebersberger, I., Riedel-Christ, S., Enders, G., Leukert, L. and Kraiczy, P., 2019. The Acinetobacter trimeric autotransporter adhesin Ata controls key virulence traits of Acinetobacter baumannii. Virulence, 10(1), pp.68-81.

[62] Penwell, W.F. and Actis, L.A., 2019. Isolation and Characterization of the Acinetobactin and Baumannoferrin Siderophores Produced by Acinetobacter baumannii. In Acinetobacter baumannii (pp. 259-270). Humana Press, New York, NY.

[63] Bohac, T.J., Fang, L., Giblin, D.E. and Wencewicz, T.A., 2019. Fimsbactin and Acinetobactin Compete for the Periplasmic Siderophore Binding Protein BauB in Pathogenic Acinetobacter baumannii. ACS chemical biology.

[64] Penwell WF, Arivett BA, Actis LA. The Acinetobacter baumannii entA gene located outside the acinetobactin cluster is critical for siderophore production, iron acquisition and virulence. PLoS One. 2012;7:e36493.

[65] Koenigs A, Stahl J, Averhoff B, et al. CipA of Acinetobacter baumannii is a novel plasminogen binding and complement inhibitory protein. J Infect Dis. 2016;213:1388-1399.

[66] Karageorgopoulos DE, Falagas ME. Current control and treatment of multidrug-resistant Acinetobacter baumannii infections. Lancet Infect Dis. 2008;8(12):751-762.

[67] Lim, S.M.S., Sime, F.B. and Roberts, J., 2019. Multidrug-resistant Acinetobacter baumannii infections: current evidence on treatment options and role of PK/PD in dose optimization. International journal of antimicrobial agents.

[68] Mizrahi, C.J., Benenson, S., Moscovici, S., Candanedo, C., Benifla, M. and Spektor, S., 2019. Combination Treatment with Intravenous Tigecycline and Intraventricular and Intravenous Colistin in Postoperative Ventriculitis Caused by Multidrug-resistant Acinetobacter baumannii. Cureus, 11(1).

[69] Tsioutis, C., Kritsotakis, E. I., Karageorgos, S. A., Stratakou, S., Psarologakis, C., Kokkini, S., et al. (2016). Clinical epidemiology, treatment and prognostic factors of extensively drug-resistant Acinetobacter baumanni ventilatorassociated pneumonia in critically ill patients. Int. J. Antimicrob. Agents 48, 492-497.

[70] Neonakis, I. K., Spandidos, D. A., and Petinaki, E. (2011). Confronting muhidrugresistant Acinetobacter baumanii: a review. Int. J. Antimierob. Agents 37, 102-109.

[71] Ayraud-Thévenot, S., Huart, C., Mimoz, O., Taouqi, M., Laland, C., Bousseau, A., et al. (2012). Control of multi-drug-resistant Acinetobacter baumannii outbreaks in an intensive care unit: feasibility and economic

impact of rapid unit closure. J. Hosp. Infect. 82, 290-292.

[72] Kaliterna, V., and Goic-Barisic, I. (2013). The ability of biofilm formation in clinical isolates of Acinetobacter baumannii belonging to two different European clones causing outbreaks in the Split University Hospital, Croatia. J. Chemother. 25, 60-62.

[73] Garnacho MJ, Dimopoulos G, Poulakou G, et al. Task force on management and prevention of Acinetobacter baumannii infections in the ICU. Intensive Care Med. 2015;41:2057-75.

[74] Guan X, He L, Hu B, et al. Laboratory diagnosis, clinical management and infection control of the infections caused by extensively drug-resistant gram-negative bacilli: a Chinese consensus statement. Clin Microbiol Infect. 2016;22:S15-25.

[75] Hu FP, Zhu DM, Wang F, et al. Resistance trends among clinical isolates in China reported from CHINET surveillance of bacterial resistance, 2005-2014. Clin Microbiol Infect. 2016;22:S9–S14.

[76] Wu X, Chavez JD, Schweppe DK, et al. In vivo protein interaction network analysis reveals porin-localized antibiotic inactivation in Acinetobacter baumannii strain AB5075. Nat Commun. 2016;7:13414.

[77] Aggarwal R, Dewan A. Comparison of nephrotoxicity of Colistin with Polymyxin B administered in currently recommended doses: a prospective study. Ann Clin Microbiol Antimicrob. 2018;17:15.

[78] Kadoyama K, Sakaeda T, Tamon A, et al. Adverse event profile of tigecycline: data mining of the public version of the U.S. Food and Drug Administration adverse event reporting system. Biol Pharm Bull. 2012;35:967-70.

[79] Xiao T, Yu W, Niu T, et al. A retrospective, comparative analysis of risk factors and outcomes in carbapenem-susceptible and carbapenem-nonsusceptible *Klebsiella pneumoniae* bloodstream infections: tigecycline significantly increases the mortality. Infect Drug Resist. 2018;11:595-606.

[80] Vrancianu CO, Gheorghe I, Czobor IB, Chifiriuc MC. Antibiotic Resistance Profiles, Molecular Mechanisms and Innovative Treatment Strategies of Acinetobacter baumannii. Microorganisms. 2020 Jun;8(6):935.

[81] Thomson JM, Bonomo RA. The threat of antibiotic resistance in Gram-negative pathogenic bacteria: β-lactams in peril!. Current opinion in microbiology. 2005 Oct 1;8(5):518-24.

[82] Liu J, Zhu F, Feng B, Zhang Z, Liu L, Wang G. Comparative efficacy and safety of combination therapy with high-dose sulbactam or colistin with additional antibacterial agents for multiple drug-resistant and extensively drug-resistant Acinetobacter baumannii infections: a systematic review and network meta-analysis. Journal of Global Antimicrobial Resistance. 2020 Sep 2.

[83] Neshani A, Sedighian H, Mirhosseini SA, Ghazvini K, Zare H, Jahangiri A. Antimicrobial peptides as a promising treatment option against Acinetobacter baumannii infections. Microbial Pathogenesis. 2020 May 5:104238.

[84] Mwangi J, Yin Y, Wang G, Yang M, Li Y, Zhang Z, Lai R. The antimicrobial peptide ZY4 combats multidrug-resistant *Pseudomonas aeruginosa* and Acinetobacter baumannii infection. Proceedings of the National Academy of Sciences. 2019 Dec 26;116(52):26516-22.

[85] Peng J, Long H, Liu W, Wu Z, Wang T, Zeng Z, Guo G, Wu J. Antibacterial mechanism of peptide Cec4 against Acinetobacter baumannii. Infection and drug resistance. 2019;12:2417.

[86] LaVergne S, Hamilton T, Biswas B, Kumaraswamy M, Schooley RT, Wooten D. Phage therapy for a multidrug-resistant Acinetobacter baumannii craniectomy site infection. InOpen forum infectious diseases 2018 Apr (Vol. 5, No. 4, p. ofy064). US: Oxford University Press.

[87] Jeon J, Park JH, Yong D. Efficacy of bacteriophage treatment against carbapenem-resistant Acinetobacter baumannii in Galleria mellonella larvae and a mouse model of acute pneumonia. BMC microbiology. 2019 Dec 1;19(1):70.

Chapter 8

Breakthrough Host Defense: UTI in Pregnant Women in Comparsion to Non-Pregnant

Muhamed Ali Al Kabe and Eman Th. Nadhaif Al-Fatlawy

Abstract

Urinary tract infections (UTIs) are common in pregnant women and provide a substantial therapeutic challenge due to the high potential of serious effects for both the mother and the baby. Pregnancy affects the urinary system physiologically, anatomically, and functionally, which can lead to infections emerging from the urethra. Unlike the general population, all pregnant women should have their urine cultures examined for bacteriuria, and any cases of asymptomatic bacteriuria should be treated, as it is a major risk factor for pyelonephritis in this group. Both the mother and the fetus should be safe from the antibiotic administered. To determine the prevalence of UTI in pregnancy in compare to non-pregnant woman in Wasit province to roll out the impact of pregnancy on the frequency of UTI. A case–control study between 2019 July and 2019 September was carried out on 30 pregnant women in compare to 30 matched non pregnant women were attending Al-Zahraa teaching hospital. A randomized (Every member of a population has the same probability of being picked for the sample, as do all possible samples of a given size) age, employment, present history, previous history, obstetric history, sex partner, frequency of sexual intercourse, and peeing frequency were all analyzed separately utilizing a plate form questioner. Urine samples, as well as a regular urine examination and urine culture, were obtained from the women who were being studied. Bacteriouria was shown to be prevalent in 13.3% of women, 16.7% of pregnant women, and 10% of non-pregnant women in this research. Asymptomatic bacteriuria in all women was 5/60 cases 8.3%. This indicates that about 16.7% of pregnant women are at risk of development of acute episode of UTI during pregnancy if they are not properly treated. In pregnant women, urinary tract infections (UTIs) are still a prevalent concern, particularly in the second trimester. During the prenatal period, urinalysis is necessary for all pregnant women. Early diagnosis and treatment of asymptomatic bacteriuria will be aided by the screening, preventing complications for both mother and child. The most prevalent risk factors for UTI during pregnancy were poor personal cleanliness, a history of UTI, diabetes mellitus, and anemia. As a result, the study suggests that pregnant women get health education on personal sanitary cleanliness, be advised not to overuse antibiotics, and undergo frequent comprehensive urine analysis.

Keywords: pregnant woman, nonpregnant women, bacteriuria, UTI, hygiene

1. Introduction

When compared to non-pregnant women, the risk of urinary tract infection (UTI) with bacteriuria increases considerably during pregnancy. Infection with bacteriuria during pregnancy has been linked to an increased risk of pyelonephritis [1]. Several physiological changes occur during normal pregnancy, including an increase in the volume of vascular and interstitial of the renal system, which results in a rise in kidney dimension of roughly 1 cm and a 30% rise in renal volume. In addition, by mid-pregnancy, around 80% of women will have dilated upper urinary tracts, ureters, pelvis, and calycle area. The right side of the body experiences dilation more frequently than the left [2]. Hydronephrosis and hydroureter, respectively, are dilations of the kidney and ureter that occur most commonly during the second trimester and last until birth. This dilation can be caused by both hormonal and mechanical factors; an increase in progesterone hormone levels causes a decrease in bladder and ureteral tone [3]. Urinary stasis was caused by mechanical causes such as gravid uterine compression paired with smooth muscle relaxation, which slowed ureter peristalsis and increased bladder volume capacity. Pregnancy-induced alterations in urine pH, osmolality, and glycosuria may further amplify bacterial growth [2]. Symptomatic infections (acute cystitis, acute pyelonephritis) occur when bacteria invade urinary tract tissues and trigger an inflammatory reaction, whereas asymptomatic bacteriuria (ASB) occurs when bacteria grow in urine without presenting symptoms of acute UTI [1]. Asymptomatic bacteriuria is more common in pregnant women than in non-pregnant women, and it is frequently underreported since diagnosis is difficult owing to the lack of particular symptoms or signs, whereas symptomatic bacteriuria creates no concerns because diagnosis and treatment are simple [1]. The most prevalent medical complication during pregnancy is urinary tract infection (UTI), which accounts for 20% of pregnancies and 10% of antepartum hospitalizations [4–6]. The most common bacterium that causes UTI in pregnant and nonpregnant women is *Escherichia coli* [7]. Preterm delivery is more common when the bacterium group B-streptococcus is infected, and when antibiotics are used often to treat UTIs caused by other organisms [8]. Other variables that contribute to an increase in UTI during pregnancy include a narrow urethra and closeness to the anus and vagina. Wesley [9] and the inability of women to completely empty their bladder. Lower socioeconomic groups have a higher incidence [9]. The risk is also reported to be increased by sexual activity and some contraceptive techniques [10]. Because of the physical link between the female urethra and the vagina, it is susceptible to damage during sexual intercourse and microorganisms being massaged up the urethra into the bladder during pregnancy/childbirth [11, 12]. Urinary tract abnormalities or stones, diabetes, immunosuppression, and a history of UTI all enhance the risk [13, 14]. It has severe consequences for both the unborn infant and the mother. Acute pyelonephritis, poor neonatal weight, and premature birth are all elevated risks, as is the risk of pre-eclampsia [1, 15], maternal anemia, hypertension, phlebitis, and thrombosis. Some bacteria can cause uterine contraction and cervix tearing by producing inflammatory mediators (phospholipase A2, arachidonic acid, and prostaglandins) [16]. Early detection and treatment of UTI has been linked to a better pregnancy outcome and a lower incidence of acute pyelonephritis, underscoring the need of screening all pregnant women regardless of symptoms. Although urine culture is regarded as the gold standard test, it takes a long time to complete. Several fast screening assays are now in use, however the data supporting their effectiveness is of poor quality. However, it has been found that combining them is a reliable option with sensitivity and specificity equivalent to urine culture. **Objective**: This study has been carried out to determine prevalence rate of urinary tract infection in pregnancy in compare to non-pregnant woman and to roll out the impact of pregnancy on the frequency of UTI.

2. Material and methods

2.1 Study design

This case–control research comprised 30 pregnant women and 30 non-pregnant women who visited Al-zahraa Teaching Hospital's outpatient clinic on a regular basis. As a result of a randomized selection (where every member of a population has an equal probability of being included in the sample and where all feasible samples of a given size have an equal probability of being chosen), selected participants were assessed individually using a plate form questioner and agreed to participate in this study for three months, starting in July and ending in September 2019.

2.2 Sampling technique and data collection

Women who visited the al-Zahraa teaching hospital's outpatient clinic, pregnant or not, were asked to provide their verbal agreement. For roughly 10 minutes, each woman was interrogated (Women who declined to participate were not questioned, and the next lady was chosen). Age, mother socioeconomic circumstances, obstetrical history, medical history, and patient complaint are all taken into account in the case history. Patients were taught how to collect urine samples in a sterile urine container under aseptic circumstances and then send them for a general urine examination. The sample was then given a name, a number, and was quickly taken to the lab for additional analysis.

2.3 Statistical analysis

Data of this study were statistically analyzed using IBM SPSS version 22.0 and descriptive statistic was used to summaries the data, like tables, figures, and measures of central tendency. Analytic statistics were used to compare between the variables. Chi-square (x2) was used, significance was assumed at $p \leq 0.05$.

2.4 Ethical aspects

The Ethical Committee of Wasit University's College of Medicine examined the study protocol and approved it.

3. Results

3.1 Description of the studied population

In this study the prevalence of bacteriuria in women was found to be 13.3%, in pregnant women 16.7% and in non-pregnant women 10%. Asymptomatic bacteriuria in all women was 5/60 cases 8.3%. This indicates that about 16.7% of pregnant women are at risk of development of acute episode of UTI during pregnancy if they are not properly treated [17, 18].

4. Discussion

In this study the prevalence of bacteriuria in women was found to be 13.3% (8/60), in pregnant women 16.7% (5/30), and in non-pregnant women 10% (3/30). Asymptomatic bacteriuria in all women was 8.3% (5/60), in pregnant women was 11.7% (4/30), and in non-pregnant women was 5% (2/30). This indicates that about

16.7% of pregnant women are at risk of development of acute episode of UTI during pregnancy if they are not properly treated. These findings are similar to that of Uncu who reported the prevalence of asymptomatic bacteriuria in pregnant women 9.3% [19]. In a study performed in turkey, the prevalence of asymptomatic bacteriuria was reported to be 8.1% [20]. The results of the present study found significantly high relation between age and bacteriuria (p = 0.00) (**Table 1**) and revealed that the bacteriuria in women was commonest in the age group 25–30 years 62.5%, and these result agreed with study by Buzayan in Libya [21], but contrast with study in Yemen that observed the bacteriuria was more in the age group 15–24 years 53.7% [22]. The difference may be due to social factors such as early age of marriage and sexual activity. There is no significant relationship between level of education and bacteriuria (p = 0.147) (**Table 2**), the prevalence of bacteriuria was 30.8% in illiterate, 18.5% in primary, 11.1% in secondary and 5.7% in university level of education However, as the level of education increases there is decrease in bacteriuria among women and these findings are similar with Samad [23]. The prevalence of bacteriuria was 14.7% in married women, and 8% in unmarried women, differences are founded apparently but no statistical difference (p = 0.562) (**Table 2**), while Krcmery et al., showed that the risk factors for bacteriuria

Bacteriuria	Cases with Bacteriuria		Cases without Bacteriuria		Total	
Age / year	NO	%	NO	%	NO	%
	X2 = 13.744 df = 4 p = 0.0001 S					
18–24	1	18.75	8	15.3	9	15.8
25–30	5	62.5	11	22.1	16	27.5
31–36	1	6.25	18	34.7	19	30.8
37–42	1	12.5	10	18.3	11	17.6
43–48	0	0	5	9.6	5	8.3
Total	8	13.3	52	86.7	60	100

Table 1.
The distribution of cases of bacteriuria according to the age of the studied groups.

Level of Education	Cases with Bacteriuria		Cases without Bacteriuria		Total	
	NO	%	NO	%	NO	%
	X2 = 5.999 df = 3 p = 0.147 N.S.					
Illiterate	2	30.8	5	69.2	7	10.8
Primary	3	18.5	11	81.5	14	22.5
Secondary	2	11.1	20	88.9	22	37.5
University	1	5.7	16	94.3	17	29.2
Marital status	X2 = 0.304 df = 1 p = 0.562 N.S.					
Married	7	14.7	40	85.3	47	100
Un married	1	8	12	92	13	100
Total	8	13.3%	52	86.7%	60	100%

Table 2.
The distribution of cases of bacteriuria in the studied population according to their education level, marital status and UTI.

in women include sexual intercourse and having a marital history [24] (**Table 3**). The bacteriuria in the pregnant women was observed more in the third trimester 21.4% than in the first trimester 6.3%, and second trimester 20%. But no significant (p = 0.423) (**Table 4**). Similar with Haddad who found that the bacteriuria was more

Bacteriuria	Symptomatic Bacteriuria		Asymptomatic Bacteriuria		Cases without Bacteriuria		Total	
	NO	%	NO	%	NO	%	NO	%
Pregnancy	X2 = 1.754 df = 2 p = 0.416 N.S.							
Pregnant	1	3.3	4	13.3	25	83.4	30	100
Non Pregnant	2	6.7	1	3.3	17	90	30	100
Total	3	5	5	8.3	52	86.7	60	100

Table 3.
The distribution of cases of bacteriuria in relation to the pregnancy and UTI conditions.

Bacteriuria	Cases with Bacteriuria		Cases without Bacteriuria		Total	
	NO	%	NO	%	NO	%
Pregnancy Trimester	X2 = 1.719 df = 2 p = 0.423 N.S.					
First Trimester	1	6.3	15	93.7	16	26.7
Second Trimester	6	20	24	80	30	50
Third Trimester	3	21.4	11	78.6	14	23.3
Total	10	16.7	50	83.3	60	100

Table 4.
The distribution of cases of bacteriuria in relation to the pregnancy age and UTI.

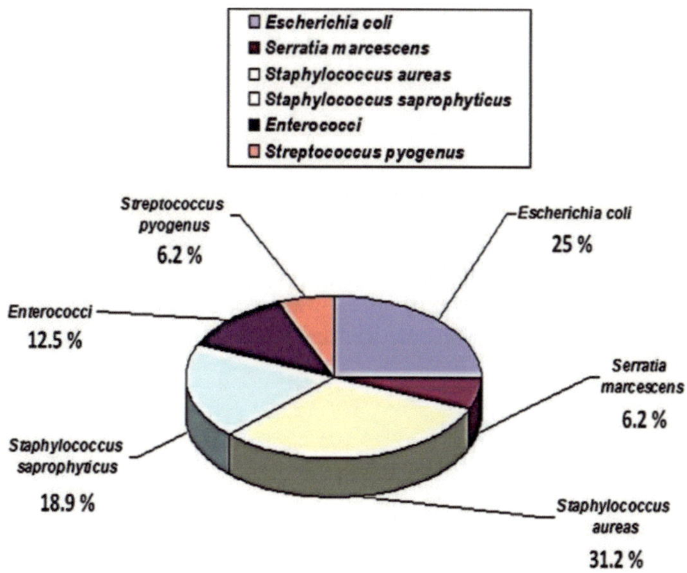

Figure 1.
The percentage of isolated bacteria responsible for bacteriuria.

in the third trimester 48.8% [22]. In contrast Buzayan [21], in this study the most frequent isolates were *Staphylococcus aureus* (31.2%), E.coli (25%), Staphylococcus saprophyticus (18.9%), Enterococcus species (12.5%), *Streptococcus pyogenes* (6.2%) and Serratia marcescens (6.2%) (**Figure 1**), whereas another Libyan study found that the bacteriuria in pregnant women caused by E.coli 65.5% and Klebsiella pneumonia 20.7% [21], and Haddad found E.coli was most frequently isolated 41.5%, followed by *Staphylococcus aureus* 19.5% [22]. The result of this study agreed with that of Oyagade et al. who found that the microbiological culture of urine samples from 502 pregnant women resulted in the isolation of bacteria, which were *Staphylococcus aureus* 21.3%, E.coli 16.0%, Staphylococcus spp. 14.7% [19]. The most effective antibiotics tested on the isolated bacteria were gentamycin (GN) 87.5%, azithromycin (AZM) 75% and ciprofloxacin (CIP) 68.75%, and the less effective antibiotics were cephalexine (CL) 6.25%, and ampicillin (AMP) 12.5%. The results of this study agreed with other studies which stated that urine culture is the gold standard method of diagnosis for bacteriuria. It's shown that urine dipstick testing, urinalysis, and enzymatic urine screening tests can poorly detect all the culture positive bacteriuria cases in women [20, 23].

5. Conclusion

The results of this work indirectly supported the hypothesis of an association of bacteriuria with age and gravidity. In addition, UTI appears to be multifactorial. A screening for bacteriuria in women especially pregnant women must be done to discover the infected cases, which would allow early treatment to avoid the complications.

6. Recommendation

The most prevalent risk factors for UTI during pregnancy were poor personal cleanliness, a history of UTI, diabetes mellitus, and anemia. The study recommends training in personal hygiene and health education about the type and frequency of changes in underwear, the number of showers per week, the use of soap, and the use of water to wash genitalia, genital dries, the frequency of micturition, precoital washing, postictal washing, and precoital micturition.

Acknowledgements

I would like to express my gratitude to the O&G seniors at the outpatient's clinic in the Al Zahraa teaching hospital for their great assistance in a achieving this research, along with al zahraa teaching hospital internal laboratory staff for their role in conducting GUE and urine culture for each participant in this study.

Author details

Muhamed Ali Al Kabe[1*] and Eman Th. Nadhaif Al-Fatlawy[2]

1 Medical Microbiology and Immunology Department, Faculty of Medicine, Wasit University, Iraq

2 Laboratory and Clinical Sciences Department, Pharmacy College, Kufa University, Iraq

*Address all correspondence to: malkaabi@uowasit.edu.iq

References

[1] Schnarr J, Smaill F. Asymptomatic bacteriuria and symptomatic urinary tract infections in pregnancy. Eur J Clin Invest 2008;38 Suppl 2:50-57.

[2] Jeyabalan A, Lain KY. Anatomic and functional changes of the upper urinary tract during pregnancy. Urol Clin North Am 2007;34:1-6.

[3] Parveen K, Momen A, Begum AA, Begum M. Prevalence of urinary tract infection during pregnancy. J Dhaka Natl Med Coll Hosp 2011;17:8-1.

[4] Alemu A, Moges F, Shiferaw Y, Tafess K, Kassu A, Anagaw B, et al. Bacterial profile and drug susceptibility pattern of urinary tract infection in pregnant women at university of Gondar Teaching Hospital, Northwest Ethiopia. BMC Res Notes 2012;5:197.

[5] Tadesse E, Teshome M, Merid Y, Kibret B, Shimelis T. Asymptomatic urinary tract infection among pregnant women attending the antenatal clinic of Hawassa Referral Hospital, Southern Ethiopia. BMC Res Notes 2014;7:155.

[6] Vasudevan R. Urinary tract infection: An overview of the infection and the associated risk factors. J Microbiol Exp 2014;1:8.

[7] Olds SB, Ladewig W, Davidson MR. Maternal Newborn Nursing and Women's Health Care. 7th ed. United States of America: New Jersey; 2004. p. 120-122.

[8] Allen VM, Yudin MH, Bouchard C, Boucher M, Caddy S, Castillo E, et al. Infectious Diseases Committee, Society of Obstetricians and Gynaecologists of Canada. Management of group B streptococcal bacteriuria in pregnancy. J Obstet Gynaecol Can 2012;34:482-486.

[9] Wesley WE. Urinary tract infection. Females Med J 2002; 3:33-41.

[10] Bandyopadhyay S, Thakur JS, Ray P, Kumar R. High prevalence of bacteriuria in pregnancy and its screening methods in North India. J Indian Med Assoc 2005; 103: 259-262, 266.

[11] Arthur LB, Smith PB, Marvin T. Clinical consideration;laboratory diagnosis of UTI. 1975;USA, 2:1-4.

[12] Duerden BI, Reid TMS, Jewsbury JM, Turk. A New Short book of Medical Parasitic Infection.DC 1990; ELBS Publishers. 576- 582.

[13] Patterson, T.F. and V.T. Andriole, Detection, significance and therapy of Bacteriuria in pregnancy; update in the managed health care era. Infect. Dis. Clin. North Am. 1997; 11: 593-608.

[14] London: WB Saunders, 1999; 559: 559-98.

[15] Bolton M, Horvath DJ Jr., Li B, Cortado H, Newsom D, White P, et al. Intrauterine growth restriction is a direct consequence of localized maternal uropathogenic Escherichia coli cystitis. PLoS One 2012; 7:e33897.

[16] Randis TM, Gelber SE, Hooven TA, Abellar RG, Akabas LH, Lewis EL, et al. Group B streptococcus β-hemolysin/cytolysin breaches maternal-fetal barriers to cause preterm birth and intrauterine fetal demise in vivo. J Infect Dis 2014; 210:265-273.

[17] Uncu Y; Uncu G; Esmer A and Bilgel N. (2002), Should asymptomatic bacteriuria be screened in pregnancy? Clin. Exp. Obstet. Gynecol. 29:281-285.

[18] Tugrul S; Oral O; Kumru P; Kose D; Alkan A and Yildirim G. (2005). Evaluation and importance of asymptomatic bacteriuria in pregnancy. Clin Exp Obstet Gynecol. 32:237-240.

[19] Oyagade AO; nSI Smith; and O Famurewaf. (2004). Asymptomatic significant bacteriuria among pregnant women in ADO-EKIT Ekit Sstate, Nigeria, African Journal of Clinical and Experimental Microbiology Vol.5, No.1.

[20] Teppa RJ and Roberts JM. (2005). The uriscreen test to detect significant asymptomatic bacteriuria during pregnancy. J Soc Gynecol Investig. 12:50-53.

[21] Buzayan Muna Mohamed. (1998) Astudy of bacteriuria during pregnancy in Benghazis women. Benghazi university. (Unpublished thesis).

[22] Al-Haddad A.M. (2005) Urinary tract infection among pregnant women, Eastern Mediterranean Health Journal, Vol 11 No 3:505- 510.

[23] Samad Hazhir. (2007) Asymptomatic bacteriuria in pregnant women, Urology Journal Vol 4 No1.

[24] Krcmery S; Hromec J and Demesova D. (2001) Treatment of lower urinary tract infection in pregnancy. Int J Antimicrob Agents, 17(4):279-282.

Chapter 9

Ureteric Injury in Gynecology Surgery

Rama Garg

Abstract

It is the most serious and trouble-some complication of pelvic surgery and common reason for medico-legal action by the patient. It can be unilateral or bilateral. Lowest 3 cm of ureter is usually injured. 75% of injuries result from gynecological operations - 3/4th during abdominal and 1/4th during vaginal operations. As most injuries can be diagnosed intraoperatively, systematic assessment of urinary tract integrity should be part of the surgical plan. Intraoperative cystoscopy using either flexible or rigid instruments can aid in the diagnosis or exclusion of urinary tract injury. Identification of the mechanism of injury and its location guides immediate or delayed repair. Mobilization should be sufficient to allow a tension-free closure. Tissue interposition is typically recommended. Common sites for ureteral injury are found beneath the uterine vessels near the cardinal ligament and beneath the infundibulopelvic ligament and the tunnel of Wertheim. Successful ureteral repair relies on careful mobilization, wide spatulation, use of fine absorbable suture (4-0, 5-0), and temporary stenting. Postoperative signs and symptoms of ureteral injury may include unilateral flank pain, fever, prolonged ileus, and abdominal or pelvic fluid collection (urinoma).

Keywords: Ureteric, Injury, Gynecology, Surgery, Prevention, Ureteroureterostomy

1. Introduction

Involuntary continuous leakage of urine after gynecological surgery comes as a bolt from blue to the patient and may cause suffering many times more than her previous disease. It is the most serious and trouble-some complication of pelvic surgery and common reason for medico-legal action by the patient [1].

2. Incidence

It can be unilateral or bilateral [1–6].

Abd. Hysterectomy	➔	0.5%-1.0%
Vaginal Hysterectomy	➔	0.1%
Adnexectomy	➔	0.1%
Extensive Hysterectomy	➔	1-2%
Laparoscopy associated ureteral injury	➔	0.3-0.4%

Lowest 3 cm of ureter is usually injured.
75% of injuries from gynecological operations.

- 3/4 during abdominal operations.
- 1/4 during vaginal operations.

3. Type/Mechanism

- Crushing from misapplication of clamp [1–6].
- ligation with suture.
- transection – partial or complete.
- angulation with secondary obstruction - partial or complete.
- ischemia from stripping of blood supply from the wall of ureter.
- resection
- Cauterization – electrical, thermal, laser and stapler injuries in laparoscopic surgery.

4. Surgical anatomy and anatomical locations

- At or below the infundibulopelvic ligament (**Figures 1–5**) [1–6].
- Along the course of ureter on the lateral pelvic side wall just above the uterosacral ligament.
- Where the ureter passes beneath the uterine vessels.
- Beyond the uterine vessels as the ureter passes through the tunnel in the cardinal ligament and turns anteriorly and medially to enter the bladder.
- Intramural portion of ureter when it traverses the bladder wall.
- Devascularization especially in the lower 1/3$^{rd.}$

5. Association with gynecological surgery

- Most common site - pelvic brim near the infundibulopelvic ligament where it is crossed by common iliac artery, is more prone to injury due to adhesions especially in endometriosis and malignancy (**Figures 4** and **5**) [1–6]
- Most common procedure - Total abdominal hysterectomy
- Most common type of injury - obstruction

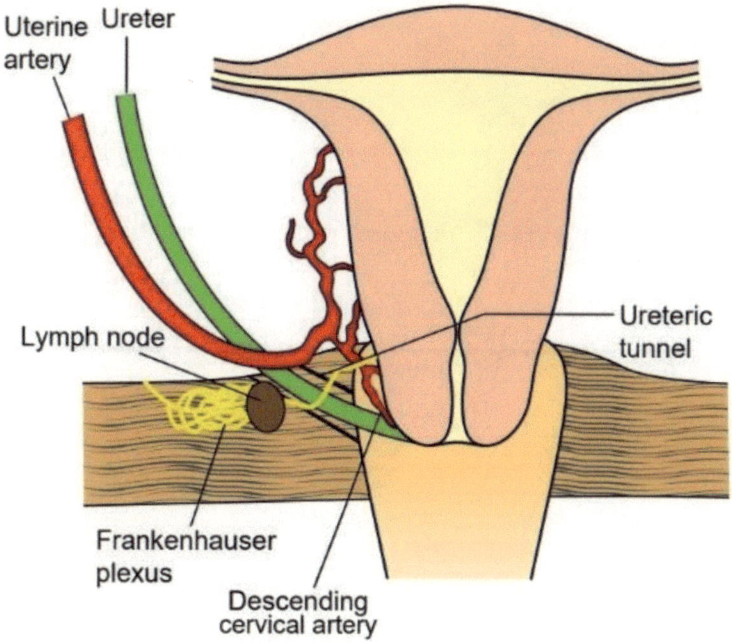

Figure 1.
Structures in the cardinal ligament—descending cervical branch of the uterine artery, ureter in the ureteric tunnel, lymph node and Frankenhauser plexus. Taken from [1].

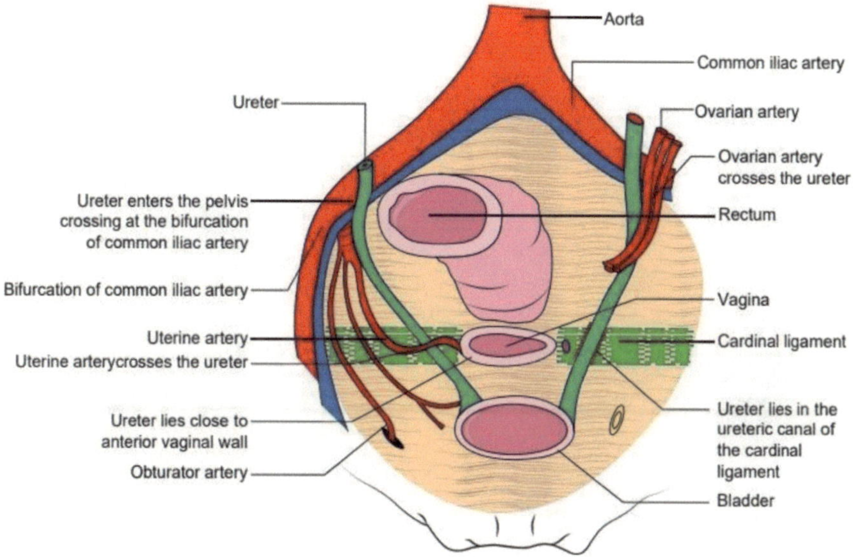

Figure 2.
Course of pelvic ureters. Taken from [1].

- Most common activity - attempts to achieve hemostasis.
- Most common time of diagnosis-None: 50-50 split between intraoperative and post-operative.
- Most common long term sequalae – None, however patient may need for repeat surgery.

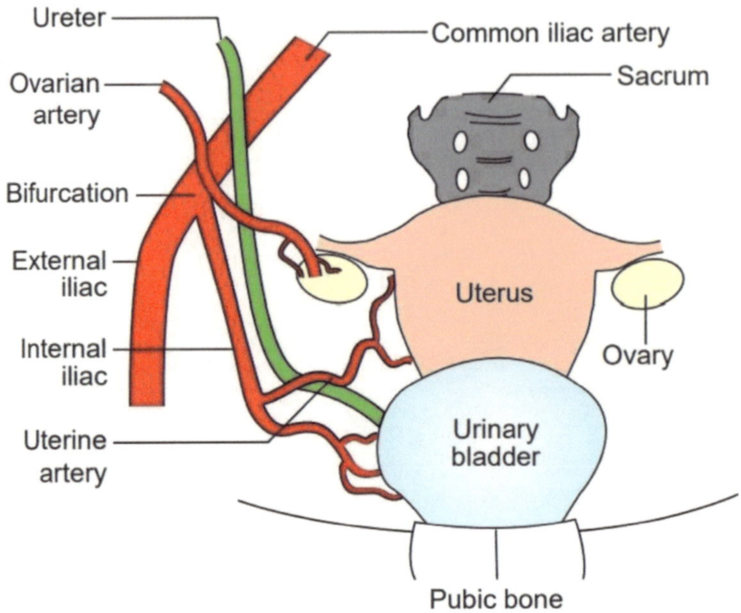

Figure 3.
Relations of the pelvic ureter. It crosses the bifurcation of vessels and then crosses under the uterine artery to enter the ureteric tunnel. Taken from [1].

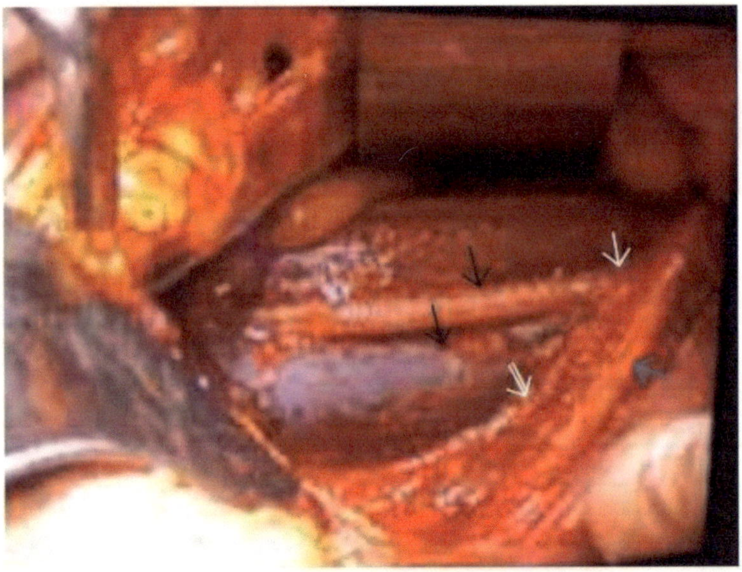

Figure 4.
Pelvic lymphadenectomy. The external iliac artery (black arrow), vein (black double arrow), bifurcation of common iliac artery (white arrow) and internal iliac artery (white double arrow). The ureter is seen crossing the common iliac at its bifurcation (blue arrow). Taken from [1].

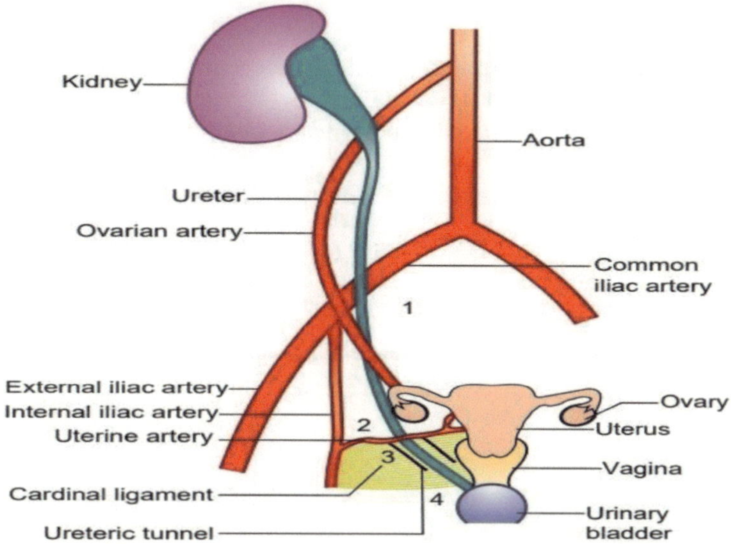

Figure 5.
Various points at which ureter is prone to injury in gynaecological surgery. (1) At the pelvic brim, while clamping the ovarian vessels. (2) In the broad ligament while clamping the uterine vessels. (3) In the ureteric tunnel in cardinal ligament. (4) At the vault of the vagina before it enters the bladder. Taken from [1].

6. Sequalae

- Spontaneous resolution and healing when injury is mild [1–6].
- Post hydronephrotic renal atrophy with complete ligation of a ureter.
    - If no sepsis ➔ asymptomatic kidney atrophy.
    - If sepsis ➔ becomes evident immediately.
- Secondary stenosis and kidney damage.
    - Ureteral necrosis with urinary extravasation
    - Ureterovaginal fistula
    - Urinoma
    - retroperitoneal abscess
    - urinary ascites (URINOMA)
    - peritonitis
- Uraemia due to bilateral ureteric obstruction ➔ flank pain, unexplained or persistent fever with or without chills, BUN and creatinine levels rise.

- Anuria for first 24-48 hours.
    - In first week ➔ Atrophy of distal nephrons.
    - In second week ➔ Atrophy of cortical region.
    - Renal Biopsy ➔ Protein casts in Bowman's space are pathognomonic of obstruction.

7. Prevention

- Primary prevention [1–6]
- Secondary prevention
- Tertiary prevention

7.1 Primary prevention

Prevention of injury before it occurs. As most injuries can be diagnosed intraoperatively, systematic assessment of urinary tract integrity should be part of the surgical plan.

Never cut/clamp /suture/apply energy before proper identification of ureter. always remember to preserve the blood supply of ureter. inadverent injury if suspected though not confirmed (blunt trauma/devascularization/ lateral damage due to thermal energy), ureteric stenting/catheterisation is to be done. always be proactive to involve the urogynaecologist at the earliest stage before, during or after surgery.

1. Careful evaluation of patient's gynecological disease and recognition of risk to the ureter with the surgical procedure is of foremost importance.

2. Preoperative excretory urogram- is mandatory in high-risk cases.

3. Ureteral catheterization by cystostomy or cystoscopically where ureter is at high risk, may be done (**Figure 6**).

4. Adequate incision and proper exposure are most helpful.

5. Ureter must not be hidden in the operator's subconscious mind - Never cut or clamp anything in and around ureter unless ureter is defined and stay outside the adventitial sheath when dissecting the ureter. Avoid energy sources near ureter especially monopolar cautery. Harmonic energy use is best near ureter next to cold scissors.

6. Before clamping infundibulopelvic ligament - surgeon must identify the ureter, lift the infundibulopelvic ligament and only then apply the clamp. First clamp should be lowest and lateral and second clamp above and medial.

7. 3 rules after skeletonization of uterine vessels

    - Place the lowest clamp first.

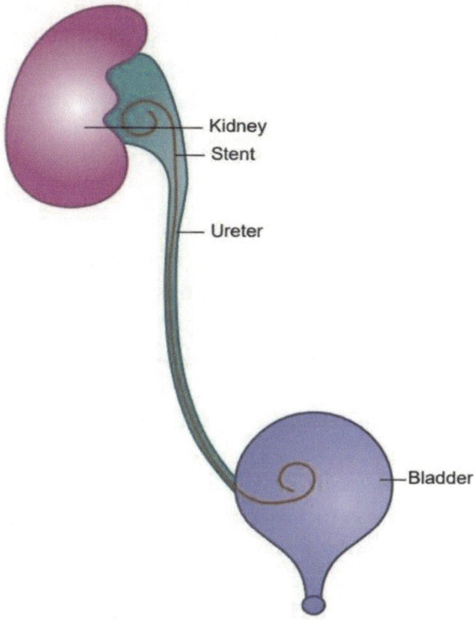

Figure 6.
Double pigtail stent placed in the ureter for management of crush injury or after repair of transection. Taken from [1].

- Place it at right angle to uterus.
- Place it at the level of internal os.
- Ligation of uterine vessels should be medial to ureter so that ureteric branch of uterine artery can be preserved.

8. Dissection of bladder from upper vagina both inferiorly and laterally is required before excising cervix from vaginal vault.

9. Paracervical and paravaginal clamps or sutures should be as close as possible to cervix.

10. To support the vault with uterosacral ligament sutures should not be placed high or more laterally on side wall otherwise ureter may get kinked or ligated.

11. Carefully reperitonise the pelvis or one may leave reperitonisation.

12. To control the intraoperative bleeding best is to apply pressure with a pack or stick sponge or finger.

13. During vaginal hysterectomy

    - vesico-uterine space must be dissected adequately to allow displacement of ureters away from the clamp by downward traction on cervix and countertraction upward beneath the bladder.
    - Small-small bits of paracervical and parametrial tissues should be clamped, cut, and ligated.

- Double clamping of cardinal ligaments and uterine vessels should be avoided as lateral clamp will come close to the ureter.

14. Perform a supracervical hysterectomy during caesarean section or extend the hysterotomy incision caudally to cervix.

15. During laparoscopic surgery:

    - If ureters are not visualized, retroperitoneal dissection should be done to decrease the incidence of complications (**Figure 4**). Visualization under Invisible near infrared (NIR) light after intravenous. or retrograde injection of ICG (Indigo carmine) dye is very useful if needed but it is expensive.

    - In tubal sterilization - Fallopian tubes should be taken away from pelvic wall before electrocoagulation.

    - In LAVH - if stapler application in cardinal and uterosacral ligament is not safe, then this part of operation should be done vaginally.

Note: Kinking is functionally similar to obstruction till it is undone. Be careful when clamping or suturing the uterosacral ligament and during reperitonisation.

7.2 Secondary prevention

Recognition of injury during operation so that immediate repair can be done. (**Figure 6–12**)

Intraoperative cystoscopy using either flexible or rigid instruments can aid in the diagnosis or exclusion of urinary tract injury. Identification of the mechanism of injury and its location guides immediate or delayed repair.

Evaluation of ureter should be done before operative procedure is terminated by:

- Inspection of peristaltic activity.

- Palpation, mobilization

- Dissection by reflecting peritoneum.

- Ureteral catheterization. (**Figure 6**)

- I/V chromogen test

- 2.5-5ml of indigo carmine 0.8% / Methylene Blue - within 3-5 minutes spurt from each ureteric orifice is there. If takes longer time - I/V fluids or diuretics are given.

- If no spurting, ureter should be explored along its course to point out the site of obstruction or injury.

- If transection is partial or complete - dye will leak into operative field.

- If ligation by suture/kinking is complete - No dye will leak in operative field and there will be proximal dilatation of ureter which will increase progressively.

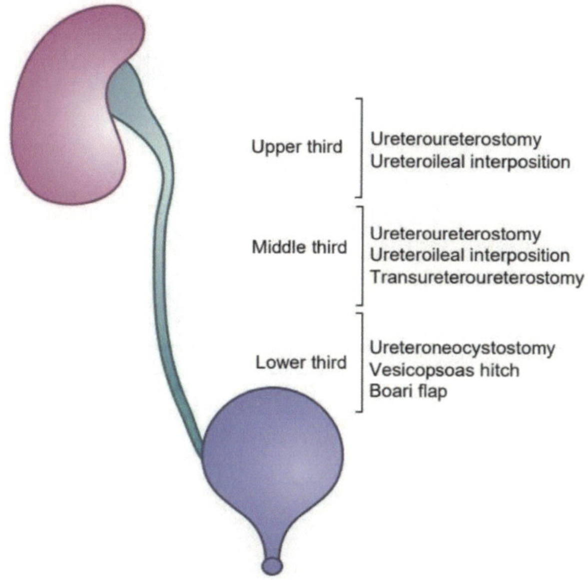

Figure 7.
Management of transection of the ureter depends on the level at which ureter is transected, that is, in the upper third, middle third or lower third. Taken from [1].

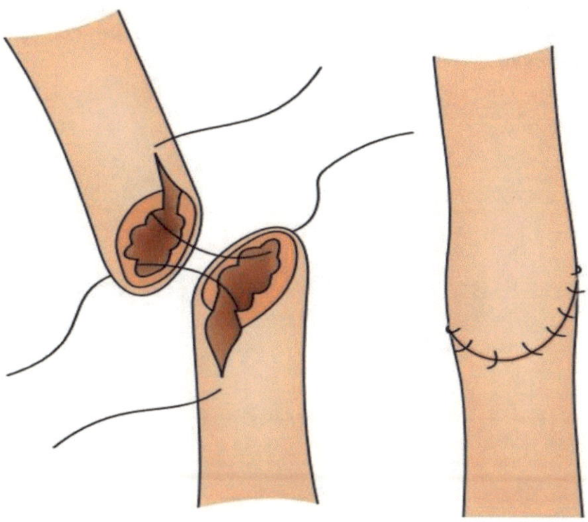

Figure 8.
Diagrammatic representation of ureteroureterostomy. The ends are spatulated and sutured. Taken from [1].

- If ligation by suture/kinking incomplete - - No dye will leak in operative field and there will be proximal dilatation of ureter that will decrease slowly and slowly.

- Intraoperative cystoscopy: Urine efflux from the ureteric orifice may be absent or slow on intraoperative cystoscopy. Almost 90% of ureteric injuries are diagnosed by cystoscopy. Partial obstruction and thermal injuries may be missed.

Note: if peristalsis seen, most probably injury is not there. but it cannot rule out ischaemic injury which will manifest postoperatibely only and may manifest after

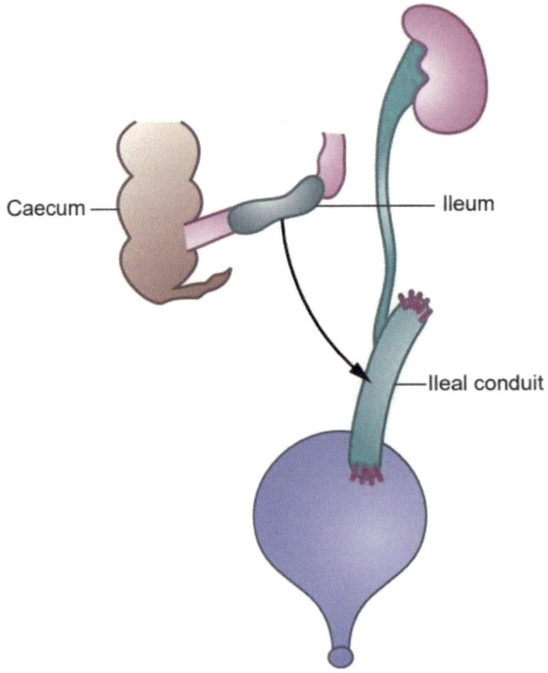

Figure 9.
Transposition of the ileum is performed when the lower segment is not long enough to implant into the bladder without tension. A distal segment of the ileum is cut and attached to the ureter at the upper end and implanted into the bladder at the lower end. Taken from [1].

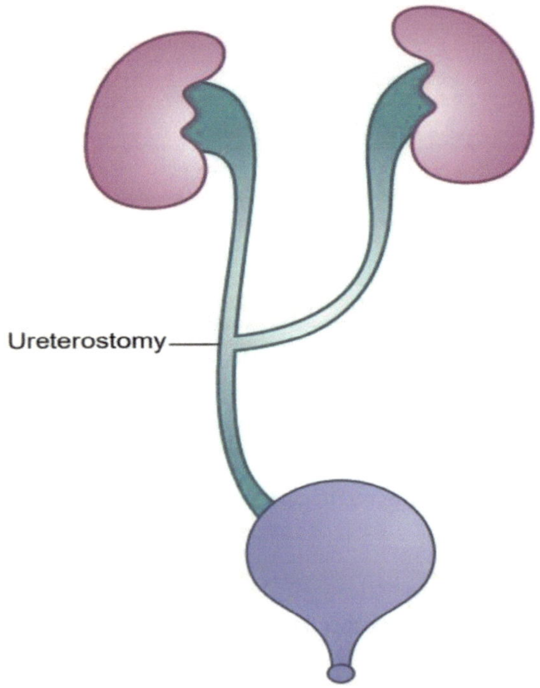

Figure 10.
Transureteroureterostomy—when the length of the lower segment of the ureter is not adequate, the cut end is anastomosed to the ureter on the opposite side. Taken from [1].

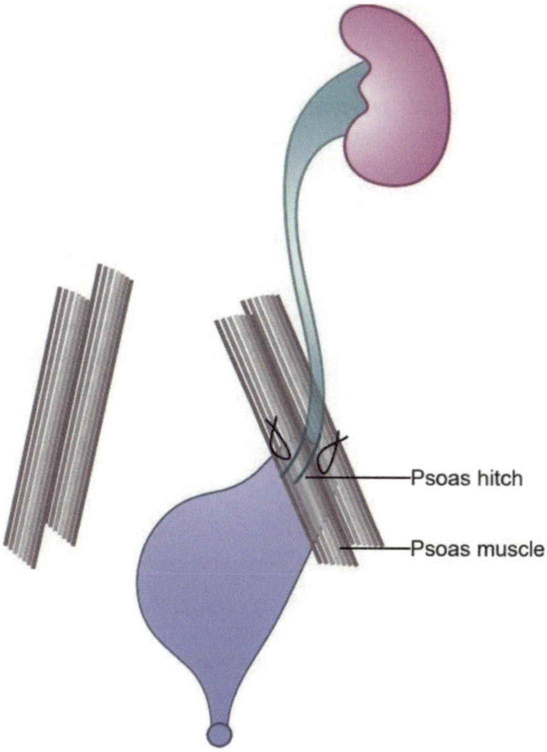

Figure 11.
A bladder flap (boari flap) shaped into a tube and the lower end of the ureter is attached to this to provide extra length and prevent tension. Taken from [1].

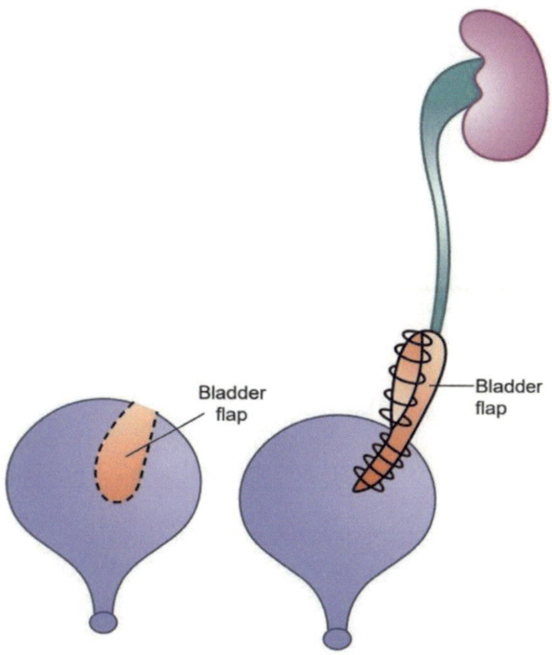

Figure 12.
Psoas hitch procedure. the bladder is pulled up and stiched to the psoas muscle to prevent tension after ureteroneocystostomy. Taken from [1].

7-10 days. so, if inadverent injury if suspected though not confirmed, ureteric stenting/catheterisation is to be done, to prevent further complications.

- Surgical procedures as per need are to be done as given under tertiary prevention depending on individual factors like site of injury, extent of damage and integrity of opposite ureter provided patient's condition allows. If unfit, temporary measures like closed drainage/PCN are taken till general condition is fit i.e., within 48-72hours or later after 6-8 weeks.

7.3 Tertiary prevention

Recognition of injury as early as possible in postoperative phase (**Figures 6–12**)
Signs/Symptoms of patient: STORMY POSTOPERATIVE PERIOD

- flank pain
- cost-vertebral tenderness
- persistent ileus
- lower abdominal mass/ ascites- Paracentesis to be done for urea level.
- unexplained fever with/without chills
- unexplained hematuria
- oliguria
- watery discharge from vagina.

8. Diagnosis

- USG may show unilateral or bilateral hydroureter or hydroureteronephrosis/ urinary ascites [1–6].
- Excretory urogram
- IV Indigo carmine test
- Pyridium/ Methylene blue test
- 3 swab tests with Methylene blue
- Cystoscopy with passage of retrograde ureteral stent, if possible, should be done.
- Comparison of pre and postoperative creatinine level.

9. Treatment depends upon

- Site of injury (distance from bladder) [1–6]
- Integrity of opposite ureter.

- Loss of length
- Time of Dx:
    - o recognized during surgery.
    - o unrecognized during surgery

9.1 General guidelines for management of ureteral injuries

This depends on the type and timing of presentation, the site of injury and the patient's condition. Immediate treatment is to relieve obstruction and stop leakage of urine. Definitive surgery for women with intraperitoneal or extraperitoneal leakage or obstruction, this should be undertaken as soon as the patient is stable and ready. Management of transaction and thermal injuries is the same as of intraoperatively diagnosed injuries. Very small fistulas may close with stenting. For large fistulas and when urine leaks despite stenting, surgery is required (**Figure** 7).

9.2 Principles

Mobilization should be sufficient to allow a tension-free closure. Tissue interposition is typically recommended. Common sites for ureteral injury are found beneath the uterine vessels near the cardinal ligament and beneath the infundibulopelvic ligament and the tunnel of Wertheim. Successful ureteral repair relies on careful mobilization, wide spatulation, use of fine absorbable suture (4-0, 5-0), and temporary stenting.

• Crushing/ Angulation/Ligation	• Deligation, assessment of vitality and stent placement (**Figure 6**)
• Partial Transection	• Primary repair over ureteral stent
• Total Transection	• Uncomplicated/ Complicated (when a segment of ureter is/has to be cut due to extensive damage)
Upper & middle third	• Ureteroureterostomy over the stent. (**Figure 8**). • Ureteroileal interposition/ Uretero-entero-neocystostomy - when an ileal segment is interposed between the two cut ends of the ureter or between the ureter and the bladder (**Figure 9**) • Transureteroureterostomy (**Figure 10**) -done occasionally only these days. • Boari flap is also used for extensive midureteral injuries. Boari bladder flap is fashioned with bladder wall; ureter is tunnelled in and attached to the flap. (**Figure 12**)
Lower third	• Uretero- neocystostomy over ureteral stent (**Figure 11**) Ureteroneocystostomy is reimplantation of ureter into the bladder. • Psoas hitch/ Vesico-psoas (**Figure 11**) In vesico-psoas hitch, the bladder is mobilized and fixed to the psoas muscle to relieve tension (psoas hitch) after uretero-neocystostomy. • Boari bladder flap (**Figure 12**)
• Thermal injury - Not rare	• Dealt as above depending upon various factors as above. The damaged part must be resected.

9.2.1 Injury recognized during surgery

- Clamp and ligature should be removed immediately (**Figures 8–12**).

- Simple pelvic closed drainage should be done.
- Intubate the ureter for 7 days by means of cystoscopy/cystotomy and retrograde catheterization of ureter with
    - Infant feeding tube - No.5
    - J-shaped stent is preferable. (**Figure 6**)
- If ureter is discovered to be cut or if extensive damage after clamping or ligation -Injury to lower third is most common
    - Injury to ureter < 4-5cm of ureterovesical junction
        - If 3–4 cm proximal to ureterovesical junction ➔ Ureteroureterostomy is needed.
        - If within 2 cm of ureterovesical junction ➔ Ureteroneocystostomy is required.
        - If above two cannot be done without tension ➔ Vesicopsoas hitch is the procedure required.
    - Injury to ureter > 4-5cm of ureterovesical junction/at brim
        - Bladder flap (Boari) (**Figure 12**)
        - Uretero-ureteral anastomosis (**Figure 8**)
        - Transperitoneal anastomosis to opposite ureter (**Figure 10**). Rarely done these days
        - Small intestine can be used as a conduit for the lower ureter-ileal conduit (**Figure 9**)
        - Skin ureterostomy

9.2.2 Injuries unrecognized during surgery

- Immediate ureteral catheterization and bypass the obstruction— should be left for 14 days or longer.
- If catheterization not possible:
    - Diagnosed within 48-72 hours of surgery- immediate ureteral repair should be done.

If diagnosis is made late or if extensive devascularization and injury are likely to occur e.g., after extensive hysterectomy, or extensive retroperitoneal fibrosis, cellulitis and induration is expected in patients with poor medical condition -PCN (Percutaneous Nephrostomy) preferably under ultrasound is required and definitive surgery can be planned 6-8 weeks later.

10. Videos

https://medicallearninghub.com/course/ureteric-safety-in-complex-gynecology-surgeries#

11. Conclusions

Sound knowledge of ureteral anatomy is critical to the avoidance of injury. In the event that the ureter is damaged during gynecologic surgery, intraoperative diagnosis allows for immediate repair in most cases. For this reason, intraoperative confirmation of ureteral integrity should be routine, whether the surgical approach is transvaginal or transabdominal through the open, laparoscopic, or robot-assisted approach. The ureter may be assessed visually, by palpation, or cystoscopically. Identification of the mechanism of injury and its location guides immediate or delayed repair. With proper recognition and therapy, ureteral function can be restored, and renal function maintained.

Acknowledgements

I am extremely grateful to my family for always being there to support me. I want to thank my parents who always believed in me. I would especially like to thank my children for constantly motivating me to work harder and my granddaughter for constantly cheering me up.

Funding

No.

Conflict of interest

The author declares no conflict of interest.

Thanks

Thank you very much Er Sidharth Garg (M Eng Electrical and Computer) for formatting the paper and making all the necessary edits to achieve its desired structure and Dr. Muskaan Bharti MBBS Intern for editing the chapter.

Author details

Rama Garg
Adesh Institute of Medical Sciences and Research, Adesh University, Bathinda, Punjab, India

*Address all correspondence to: drramagarg@gmail.com

References

[1] Seshadri L. Essentials of Gynaecology. 2 ed. Wolters Kluwer Health (India); 2019. 11,12,386-393 p. ISBN-13: 978-93-5129-698-0 www.wolterskluwerindia.co.in

[2] Victoria L. Handa, Linda Van Le. Te Linde's Operative Gynecology. 12th ed. Wolters Kluwer; 2020. 460-462,461f,633-649,649f p. Indian Reprint ISBN-13: 978-93-89702-84-2. Original ISBN-13: 9781496386441

[3] Marcus E. Setchell, John H. Shepherd, Christopher N. Hudson. Shaw's Textbook of Operative Gynaecology. 7th ed. Elsevier India; 2013. 17, 372,383-389 p. ISBN: 978-81-312-1160-1

[4] Kumar S, editor. Howkins & Bourne, Shaw's Textbook of Gynecology 17th ed. ELSEVIER; 2019. 23-25,377-384 p. ISBN: 978-81-312-5411-0. e-Book ISBN: 978-81-312-5412-7

[5] Kumar P, Malhotra N, editors. JEFFCOATE'S PRINCIPLES OF GYNAECOLOGY. 7th International ed. Jaypee Brothers Medical Publishers (P) Ltd 2008. 41,263-268,778 p. ISBN: 978-81-8448-288-1 Visit our website: www.jaypeebrothers.com

[6] Konar H, editor. DC Dutta's Textbook of Gynecology. 7th ed. Jaypee Brothers Medical Publishers (P) Ltd; 2016. 11-12,345,349-51 p. ISBN 978-93-85891-59-5 www.jaypeebrothers.com